# Natural Feed Additives and Novel Approaches for Healthy Rabbit Breeding

# Natural Feed Additives and Novel Approaches for Healthy Rabbit Breeding

Editors

**Iveta Plachá**
**Monika Pogány Simonová**
**Andrea Lauková**

MDPI • Basel • Beijing • Wuhan • Barcelona • Belgrade • Manchester • Tokyo • Cluj • Tianjin

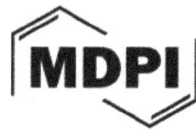

*Editors*
Iveta Plachá
Centre of Biosciences of the
Slovak Academy of Sciences
Slovakia

Monika Pogány Simonová
Centre of Biosciences of the
Slovak Academy of Sciences
Slovakia

Andrea Lauková
Centre of Biosciences of the
Slovak Academy of Sciences
Slovakia

*Editorial Office*
MDPI
St. Alban-Anlage 66
4052 Basel, Switzerland

This is a reprint of articles from the Special Issue published online in the open access journal *Animals* (ISSN 2076-2615) (available at: https://www.mdpi.com/journal/animals/special_issues/Healthy_Rabbit_Breeding).

For citation purposes, cite each article independently as indicated on the article page online and as indicated below:

LastName, A.A.; LastName, B.B.; LastName, C.C. Article Title. *Journal Name* **Year**, *Volume Number*, Page Range.

**ISBN 978-3-0365-5749-6 (Hbk)**
**ISBN 978-3-0365-5750-2 (PDF)**

© 2022 by the authors. Articles in this book are Open Access and distributed under the Creative Commons Attribution (CC BY) license, which allows users to download, copy and build upon published articles, as long as the author and publisher are properly credited, which ensures maximum dissemination and a wider impact of our publications.

The book as a whole is distributed by MDPI under the terms and conditions of the Creative Commons license CC BY-NC-ND.

# Contents

**Iveta Placha, Monika Pogány Simonová and Andrea Lauková**
Natural Feed Additives and Novel Approaches for Healthy Rabbit Breeding
Reprinted from: *Animals* **2022**, *12*, 2111, doi:10.3390/ani12162111 . . . . . . . . . . . . . . . . . . **1**

**Yordan Martínez, Maidelys Iser, Manuel Valdivié, Manuel Rosales, Esther Albarrán and David Sánchez**
Dietary Supplementation with *Agave tequilana* (Weber Var. Blue) Stem Powder Improves the Performance and Intestinal Integrity of Broiler Rabbits
Reprinted from: *Animals* **2022**, *12*, 1117, doi:10.3390/ani12091117 . . . . . . . . . . . . . . . . . . **5**

**Monika Pogány Simonová, Ľubica Chrastinová, Jana Ščerbová, Valentína Focková, Iveta Plachá, Zuzana Formelová, Mária Chrenková and Andrea Lauková**
Preventive Potential of Dipeptide Enterocin A/P on Rabbit Health and Its Effect on Growth, Microbiota, and Immune Response
Reprinted from: *Animals* **2022**, *12*, 1108, doi:10.3390/ani12091108 . . . . . . . . . . . . . . . . . . **15**

**Katarzyna Roman, Martyna Wilk, Piotr Ksiażek, Katarzyna Czyż and Adam Roman**
The Effect of the Season, the Maintenance System and the Addition of Polyunsaturated Fatty Acids on Selected Biological and Physicochemical Features of Rabbit Fur
Reprinted from: *Animals* **2022**, *12*, 971, doi:10.3390/ani12080971 . . . . . . . . . . . . . . . . . . **27**

**Mahmoud A. Elazab, Ayman M. Khalifah, Abdelmotaleb A. Elokil, Alaa E. Elkomy, Marwa M. Rabie, Abdallah Tageldein Mansour and Sabrin Abdelrahman Morshedy**
Effect of Dietary Rosemary and Ginger Essential Oils on the Growth Performance, Feed Utilization, Meat Nutritive Value, Blood Biochemicals, and Redox Status of Growing NZW Rabbits
Reprinted from: *Animals* **2022**, *12*, 375, doi:10.3390/ani12030375 . . . . . . . . . . . . . . . . . . **49**

**Paola Cremonesi, Giulio Curone, Filippo Biscarini, Elisa Cotozzolo, Laura Menchetti, Federica Riva, Maria Laura Marongiu, Bianca Castiglioni, Olimpia Barbato, Albana Munga, Marta Castrica, Daniele Vigo, Majlind Sulce, Alda Quattrone, Stella Agradi and Gabriele Brecchia**
Dietary Supplementation with Goji Berries (*Lycium barbarum*) Modulates the Microbiota of Digestive Tract and Caecal Metabolites in Rabbits
Reprinted from: *Animals* **2022**, *12*, 121, doi:10.3390/ani12010121 . . . . . . . . . . . . . . . . . . **63**

**Kristina Bacova, Karin Zitterl Eglseer, Gesine Karas Räuber, Lubica Chrastinova, Andrea Laukova, Margareta Takacsova, Monika Pogany Simonova and Iveta Placha**
Effect of Sustained Administration of Thymol on Its Bioaccessibility and Bioavailability in Rabbits
Reprinted from: *Animals* **2021**, *11*, 2595, doi:10.3390/ani11092595 . . . . . . . . . . . . . . . . . . **81**

**Egon Andoni, Giulio Curone, Stella Agradi, Olimpia Barbato, Laura Menchetti, Daniele Vigo, Riccardo Zelli, Elisa Cotozzolo, Maria Rachele Ceccarini, Massimo Faustini, Alda Quattrone, Marta Castrica and Gabriele Brecchia**
Effect of Goji Berry (*Lycium barbarum*) Supplementation on Reproductive Performance of Rabbit Does
Reprinted from: *Animals* **2021**, *11*, 1672, doi:10.3390/ani11061672 . . . . . . . . . . . . . . . . . . **91**

**Iveta Placha, Kristina Bacova and Lukas Plachy**
Current Knowledge on the Bioavailability of Thymol as a Feed Additive in Humans and Animals with a Focus on Rabbit Metabolic Processes
Reprinted from: *Animals* **2022**, *12*, 1131, doi:10.3390/ani12091131 . . . . . . . . . . . . . . . . . . **107**

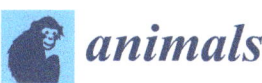 

*Editorial*

# Natural Feed Additives and Novel Approaches for Healthy Rabbit Breeding

Iveta Placha *, Monika Pogány Simonová and Andrea Lauková

Centre of Biosciences of the Slovak Academy of Sciences, Institute of Animal Physiology, Soltesovej 4-6, 040 01 Kosice, Slovakia
* Correspondence: placha@saske.sk; Tel.: +421-55-792-2969

Rabbit meat offers excellent nutritive and dietetic properties, but digestive disturbances, mainly during the post-weaning period, induce important economic losses for rabbit farmers. Recently, many studies have focused on feed additives which are able to improve the intestinal health and productivity of broiler rabbits. The main objectives of animal agriculture production are to produce safe food products, eliminating antibiotics with a low impact on environmental pollution. A great deal of interest has been expressed for safe and natural rabbit food with increased nutritional value without inducing bacterial resistance and potential side effects for animals. Natural feed additives such as prebiotics, beneficial microorganisms, organic acids, bacteriocins, and phytogenic compounds are able to match these requirements and can satisfy the increasing consumers' demand for natural substances; however, because they represent novel valuable substances, their research is an ongoing discipline.

This Special Issue covers a total of eight articles, including seven original studies and one review, with a focus on the effects of natural substances, bioactive compounds, and bacteriocins/enterocins on rabbit production, performance, gastrointestinal microbiota, intestinal immunity and morphology, health parameters, and metabolic processes in rabbits.

Martinez et al. [1] evaluated the effect of *Agave tequilana* stem powder on the growth performance and the intestinal integrity in broiler rabbits, and confirmed the beneficial biological activities of polyphenols and saponins, the main secondary metabolites of this plant. Obtained results justified the utilization of agave powder in rabbit production.

Pogány Simonová et al. [2] tested the preventive effect of a dipeptide enterocin $A/P$, produced by *Enterococcus faecium* (Ent) EK13 strain against the methicillin-resistant *Staphylococcus epidermidis* SE P3/Tr2a strain in a rabbit model, determining its effect on the growth performance, phagocytic activity, concentration of secretory immunoglobulin IgA, and gut microbial composition. Good health and increased weight gain reflect the beneficial effect of Ent $A/P$ on the growth performance of rabbits. The obtained results also showed that the methicillin-resistant *S. epidermidis* SE P3/Tr2a strain did not have any pathogenic effect on rabbits' health status. The preventive effect of Ent $A/P$ was recorded due to improved zootechnical parameters, stimulated non-specific immunity, and the stabilized intestinal microbial environment of rabbits.

Roman et al. [3] demonstrated the impact of environmental conditions (laboratory, summer and winter; and outdoor, summer and winter); and dietary supplementation with ethyl esters of linseed oil on the quality of rabbit coat hair. The environmental conditions had a considerable impact on the quality of the rabbit coat; the best results of hair thickness and their heat protection were obtained during the outdoor period. The administration of linseed oil ethyl esters had a positive effect on the hair fatty acids profile; increases in omega-3 acids and decreases in the ratio of omega-6 to omega-3 acids were observed.

Elazab et al. [4] focused their attention on the use of phytogenic feed additives, essential oils (EOs) of rosemary and ginger, as environmentally friendly supplementation

**Citation:** Placha, I.; Pogány Simonová, M.; Lauková, A. Natural Feed Additives and Novel Approaches for Healthy Rabbit Breeding. *Animals* 2022, *12*, 2111. https://doi.org/10.3390/ani12162111

Received: 9 August 2022
Accepted: 15 August 2022
Published: 17 August 2022

**Publisher's Note:** MDPI stays neutral with regard to jurisdictional claims in published maps and institutional affiliations.

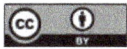

**Copyright:** © 2022 by the authors. Licensee MDPI, Basel, Switzerland. This article is an open access article distributed under the terms and conditions of the Creative Commons Attribution (CC BY) license (https://creativecommons.org/licenses/by/4.0/).

to improve rabbit growth performance, feed utilization, meat nutritive value, physiological, and redox status. The authors recommended both EOs for improving sustainable production in the rabbit industry, seeing that body weight gain and feed conversion ratio were improved; cholesterol level in muscle and plasma, as well as triglycerides in plasma, were significantly reduced; muscle fat was decreased; and the oxidant/antioxidant balance was attenuated.

Cremonesi et al. [5] investigated the effect of goji berry, the fruits of the *Lycium barbarum* plant used in traditional Chinese medicine, on the microbiota composition of different parts of the rabbit digestive tract. The obtained results suggested that goji berries could modulate the microbiota by increasing the growth of bacterial families, such as Ruminococcaceae, Lachnospiracae, Lactobacillaceae, and particularly, the genus *Lactobacillus*. To use goji berries as innovative feeds for rabbits, the authors suggested that further studies should evaluate their impact on productive performance, gut immune system maturation, as well as resistance to gastrointestinal disorders.

Bacova et al. [6] showed that to establish suitable concentrations of phytoadditives for a beneficial effect on animal health, metabolic processes of plant compounds in animal organisms should be understood at the molecular level. The metabolic path of thymol, a major constituent of *Thymus vulgaris* L., in the rabbit organism was determined for the first time in their study. The intensive absorption of thymol from the gastrointestinal tract, its metabolism and accumulation in the kidney, and intensive metabolic and excretion processes in the liver were observed. As a consequence of thymol conversion into hydrophilic metabolite and grater elimination in the rabbit organism, thymol was only found in trace amounts in fat and muscle tissues.

Andoni et al. [7] evaluated the effect of goji berry supplementation on the reproductive and productive performance of rabbits. The authors suggested that integration with goji berry in the rabbit diet at 1% affects the reproductive activity, influencing the pattern secretion of luteinizing hormone as well as the sexual receptivity and the productive performance, inducing higher milk production in rabbit does.

A comprehensive review by Placha et al. [8] provides general information on the therapeutic and preventive effect of thymol on various human and animal diseases, followed by its bioavailability in human and animal organisms. Information from this review concerning the mode of action of thymol in animals could also be applied to human medicine and may help in the utilization of herbal medicine in human and veterinary healthcare.

The papers collected in this Special Issue not only present data on the beneficial effects of natural feed additives in rabbit nutrition, but represent the available scientific information regarding the urgent need for more studies to understand the metabolic processes of natural substances on a molecular level, to establish the beneficial dose. The obtained information could be useful for researchers, the veterinary sector, and pharmaceutical industries.

**Funding:** This research received no external funding.

**Conflicts of Interest:** The authors declare no conflict of interest.

## References

1. Martinez, Y.; Iser, M.; Valdivié, M.; Rosales, M.; Albaraán, E.; Sánchez, D. Dietary supplementation with *Agave tequilqna* (Weber Var. Blue) stem powder improves the performance and intestinal integrity of broiler rabbits. *Animals* **2022**, *12*, 1117. [CrossRef] [PubMed]
2. Pogány Simonová, M.; Chrastinová, Ľ.; Ščerbová, J.; Focková, V.; Plachá, I.; Formelová, Z.; Chrenková, M.; Lauková, A. Preventive potential of dipeptide Enterocine A/P on rabbit health and its effect on growth, microbiota, and immune response. *Animals* **2022**, *12*, 1108. [CrossRef] [PubMed]
3. Roman, K.; Wilk, M.; Książek, P.; Czyż, K.; Roman, A. The Effect of the Season, the Maintenance System and the Addition of Polyunsaturated Fatty Acids on Selected Biological and Physicochemical Features of Rabbit Fur. *Animals* **2022**, *12*, 971. [CrossRef] [PubMed]
4. Elazab, M.A.; Khalifah, A.M.; Elokil, A.A.; Elkomy, A.E.; Rabie, M.M.; Mansour, A.T.; Morshedy, S.A. Effect of dietary rosemary and ginger essential oils on the growth performance, feed utilization, meat nutritive value, blood biochemicals, and redox status of growing NZW rabbits. *Animals* **2022**, *12*, 375. [CrossRef] [PubMed]

5. Cremonesi, P.; Curone, G.; Biscarini, F.; Cotozzolo, E.; Menchetti, L.; Riva, F.; Marongiu, M.L.; Castiglioni, B.; Barbato, O.; Munga, A.; et al. Dietary supplementation with goji berries (*Lycium barbarum*) modulates the microbiota of digestive tract and caecal metabolites in rabbits. *Animals* **2022**, *12*, 121. [CrossRef] [PubMed]
6. Bacova, K.; Zitterl Eglseer, K.; Karas Räuber, G.; Chrastinova, L.; Laukova, A.; Takacsova, M.; Pogany Simonova, M.; Placha, I. Effect of sustained administration of thymol on its bioaccessibility and bioavailability in rabbits. *Animals* **2021**, *11*, 2595. [CrossRef] [PubMed]
7. Andoni, E.; Curone, G.; Agradi, S.; Barbato, O.; Menchetti, L.; Vigo, D.; Zelli, R.; Cotozzolo, E.; Ceccarini, M.R.; Faustini, M.; et al. Effect of goji berry (*Lycium barbarum*) supplementation on reproductive performance of rabbit does. *Animals* **2022**, *11*, 1672. [CrossRef] [PubMed]
8. Placha, I.; Bacova, K.; Plachy, L. Current knowledge on the bioavailability of thymol as a feed additive in humans and animals with a focus on rabbit metabolic processes. *Animals* **2022**, *12*, 1131. [CrossRef] [PubMed]

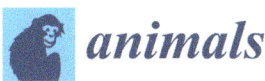

Article

# Dietary Supplementation with *Agave tequilana* (Weber Var. Blue) Stem Powder Improves the Performance and Intestinal Integrity of Broiler Rabbits

Yordan Martínez [1,*], Maidelys Iser [2], Manuel Valdivié [3], Manuel Rosales [2], Esther Albarrán [2] and David Sánchez [2]

[1] Agricultural Science and Production Department, Zamorano University, Valle de Yeguare, San Antonio de Oriente, Francisco Morazan, P.O. Box 93, Tegucigalpa 11101, Honduras

[2] Centro Universitario de Ciencias Biológicas y Agropecuarias (CUCBA), Universidad de Guadalajara, P.O. Box 49, Guadalajara 44214, Jalisco, Mexico; sofiaizabellamai@gmail.com (M.I.); manuel.rcortes@academicos.udg.mx (M.R.); esther.albarran@academsicos.udg.mx (E.A.); david.schipres@academicos.udg.mx (D.S.)

[3] National Center for Laboratory Animal Production, Santiago de las Vegas, Rancho Boyeros, La Habana P.O. Box 6240, Cuba; mvaldivie@ica.co.cu

* Correspondence: ymartinez@zamorano.edu; Tel.: +504-944422496

**Simple Summary:** Natural products have been used as an alternative to the indiscriminate use of subtherapeutic antibiotics for improving the growth of animals. Although these synthetic products have been used in rabbits to a lesser extent than in other monogastrics, several natural products have been tested with positive responses in growth performance, immune activity, and antioxidant capacity. Agaves are plants with chemical compounds that have shown positive effects on performance and animal health. Specifically, the *Agave tequilana* stem has a high content of fructans and secondary metabolites, such as polyphenols and saponins, that are responsible for various biological activities. The dietary use of up to 1.5% of *Agave tequilana* stem powder in the diet of rabbits had a natural growth-promoting effect due to the improvement of their intestinal integrity (with an emphasis on the concentric layers, villi, and crypts), taken as indicator of intestinal health. Considering the results of this study and others carried out by this group of authors, this natural product (*A. tequilana*) could be utilized in rabbit farming, considering that the stem of the agave is currently not utilized for anything.

**Abstract:** This study evaluated the effect of *Agave tequilana* (Weber var. azul) stem powder on the growth performance and the intestinal integrity in rabbits. A total of 120 male rabbits [New Zealand × California] were weaned for 35 days and randomized into four dietary treatments, 15 replicates per treatment, and two rabbits per replicate. The treatments consisted of a basal diet (T0) and dietary supplementation with 0.5% (T1), 1.0% (T2) and 1.5% (T3) of *Agave tequilana* stem powder. The T3 treatment improved the body weight and average daily gain ($p < 0.05$) compared to the other groups, without affecting viability and feed conversion ratio ($p > 0.05$). Furthermore, the T3 treatment enhanced ($p < 0.05$) the thickness of the muscular and mucous layers, and the height, thickness, and number of villi in the duodenum ($p < 0.05$). However, this treatment (T3) significantly decreased ($p < 0.05$) values for the area and depth of the crypts in the duodenum and the villus/crypt ratio. Likewise, in the cecum, T3 treatment provoked a marked decrease ($p < 0.05$) in the depth and thickness of the crypts. The results indicate that the dietary use with 1.5% of *A. tequilana* stem powder had a natural growth-promoting effect and enhanced the histomorphometry of the concentric layers (muscle and mucosa), villi, and crypts as indicators of intestinal health in rabbits.

**Keywords:** agave; intestinal mucosa; natural products; rabbit

**Citation:** Martínez, Y.; Iser, M.; Valdivié, M.; Rosales, M.; Albarrán, E.; Sánchez, D. Dietary Supplementation with *Agave tequilana* (Weber Var. Blue) Stem Powder Improves the Performance and Intestinal Integrity of Broiler Rabbits. *Animals* 2022, 12, 1117. https://doi.org/10.3390/ani12091117

Academic Editors: Iveta Plachá, Monika Pogány Simonová and Andrea Lauková

Received: 9 March 2022
Accepted: 19 April 2022
Published: 27 April 2022

**Publisher's Note:** MDPI stays neutral with regard to jurisdictional claims in published maps and institutional affiliations.

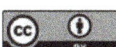

**Copyright:** © 2022 by the authors. Licensee MDPI, Basel, Switzerland. This article is an open access article distributed under the terms and conditions of the Creative Commons Attribution (CC BY) license (https://creativecommons.org/licenses/by/4.0/).

## 1. Introduction

The constant consumption of synthetic antimicrobials causes the presence of chemical residues in products of animal origin, which directly affects human health [1]. Although preventive antibiotics have been used more in poultry and pig production than in rabbit production, some reports have focused on controlling the population of *Enterobacteriaceae* with bacitracin Zn [2]. Thus, organic acids, prebiotics, probiotics, and medicinal plants have been used efficiently as viable alternatives to replace or decrease the indiscriminate use of growth-promoting antibiotics [3].

In animals, studies are carried out with natural products to evaluate intestinal health indicators, which are important for justifying the growth-promoting effect and the bactericidal, anti-inflammatory and antioxidant activities of these foods—three key considerations for nutraceuticals [4]. Furthermore, intestinal integrity, pH, and gut microbiology are known to be specifically influenced by diet and gut health [5]. In this sense, dietary use of nutraceutical products such as prebiotics and probiotics can increase the height of the villi in the small intestine, without changing the crypts depth and the natural promotion of growth in farm animals [6–9].

Plants of the genus Agaves have been used by the inhabitants of Mesoamerica for 9000 years, especially in Mexico where it originated. Of the 310 reported species, 272 of them are endemic to Mexico [10]. Among the most recognized and economically important species is the *Agave tequilana* Weber var. azul [11]. Agaves are plants with a high content of fructans synthesized and stored in the stems, and made up of polymers of fructose derived from the sucrose molecule and with glucose as a terminal monomer (generally). Moreover, the structure of fructans is used as a taxonomic marker in agaves. Specifically, the stem of the *Agave tequilana* Weber var. azul has mainly β (2→1) fructooligosaccharide linkages; and some ramifications of β (2→6) are considered to be a very complex chemical structure whose quantification will depend on the plant material (*Agave* spp.) under study [12]. Due to the high levels of fructans in *Agave tequilana*, prebiotic nutraceutical products have been obtained for their dietary use in human beings and animals [13].

Studies on farm animals reported that *Agave tequilana* stem powder acted as a natural growth promoter in diets by increasing the population of beneficial cecal bacteria and by modifying harmful serum lipids in pigs and poultry [14,15]. Likewise, authors such as Iser et al. [16] and Iser et al. [17] have demonstrated that dietary supplementation of up to 1.5% *Agave tequilana* stem powder increased productivity and meat quality, decreased harmful serum lipids, and left blood indicators of fattening rabbits unchanged. However, the study of how *A. tequilana* stem powder influences intestinal histomorphology as indicators of intestinal health could justify the growth-promoting effect of this natural prebiotic in rabbit farming. Therefore, the objective of this experiment was to evaluate the performance and histo-morphometry of the concentric layers (muscle and mucosa), villi, and crypts of the duodenum and cecum in broiler rabbits fed with supplementations of *Agave tequilana* (Weber var. Azul) powder.

## 2. Materials and Methods

### 2.1. Experimental Location

The experiment with the name CINV.106/12 was approved by the Animal Care Committee of the Faculty of Veterinary Medicine and Zootechnics of the University Center for Biological and Agricultural Sciences, University of Guadalajara (CUCBA), Mexico. It should be noted that the Mexican animal welfare guidelines and the experimental protocol were followed. The animals were housed in an open shed, and temperature (21 °C ± 2) and relative humidity (63% ± 2) were measured daily using a hygro-thermometer (Jumbo Dig).

### 2.2. Animals, Treatments, Experimental Conditions, and Diets

From a total of 350 rabbits, 120 male rabbits (New Zealand × California) that had been weaned for 35 days were selected and randomized into 4treatments, 15 replicates per treatment, and 2 rabbits per cage. The experimental treatments consisted of a basal diet formulated according to the nutritional requirements of the species under study (T0) and dietary supplementation with 0.5% (T1), 1.0% (T2), and 1.5% (T3) of *Agave tequilana* stem powder. This natural product was offered by the Veterinary Division of the *Centro Universitario de Ciencias Biológicas y Agropecuarias* (CUCBA), University of Guadalajara, Mexico. The product has the following ingredients: 93.15% dry matter; 5.08% crude protein; 1.38% crude fat; 5.15% ash; 15.98% neutral detergent fiber; 7.70% acid detergent fiber; 8.28% cellulose; and 43.24% fructans (inulin type), according to AOAC 2001.11 [18], Van Soest et al. [19], and high-performance liquid chromatography (HPLC Varian ProStar System, Palo Alto, CA, USA). Supplementation levels from a previous experiment by Iser et al. [17] were also considered for this experiment. A basal diet was prepared according to the nutritional requirements reported by Blas and Mateos [20] for fattening rabbits (Table 1).

**Table 1.** Ingredients and nutritional contributions of the diet for broiler rabbits (35 to 95 days old).

| Ingredients | Basal Diet (%) |
|---|---|
| Wheat straw | 17.4 |
| Alfalfa hay | 12.0 |
| Barleycorn | 19.0 |
| Wheat bran | 24.0 |
| Sunflower meal | 12.0 |
| Soymeal | 11.0 |
| Soy oil | 2.88 |
| Sodium chlorine | 0.50 |
| Monocalcium phosphate | 0.50 |
| L-lysine | 0.09 |
| L-threonine | 0.08 |
| DL-methionine | 0.05 |
| Premix [1] | 0.50 |
| Calculated nutritional contributions | |
| Crude protein (%) | 16.70 |
| Digestible energy (MJ/kg) | 9.92 |
| Neutral detergent fiber (%) | 35.78 |
| Detergent acid fiber (%) | 19.21 |
| Lysine (%) | 0.77 |
| Methionine + cystine (%) | 0.59 |
| Threonine (%) | 0.65 |
| Ashes (%) | 5.37 |

[1] Each kg contains: vitamin A 12,000 IU, vitamin D3 2000 IU, vitamin B2 4160 IU, Niacin 16,700 IU, pantothenic acid 8200 IU, vitamin B6 3420 IU, folic acid 0.980 g, vitamin B12 16 mg, vitamin K 1560 IU, Vitamin E 16 g, BHT 8.5 g, cobalt 0.750 g, copper 3.5 g, iron 9.86 g, manganese 6.52 g, sodium 0.870 g, zinc 4.24 g, and selenium 6.67 g.

The *A. tequilana* stem powder was added homogeneously to the mash feed, and the mixture obtained was pelleted using a rotary pelletizer (Macreat, LDS-300, Zhengzhou, China) with a particle size of 2.5 mm as established for this animal species [20].

The broiler rabbits were placed in metal cages with dimensions of 76 cm long, 76 cm wide, and 45 cm high. In two frequencies at 7:00 a.m. and 4:00 p.m., feed was supplied ad libitum, tubular galvanized sheet feeders were used, and availability adjustments were made based on the difference between supply and rejection according to Iser et al. [16]. Moreover, automatic nipple drinkers were used to offer *ad libitum* water to the rabbits.

*2.3. Growth Performance*

During the study, body weight (BW) was determined at the beginning (35 days) and at the end (95 days) of the experiment using an OSBORNE® (model 37473®, Kansas, MI, USA) digital scale with a precision of ±0.1 g. Overall mortality was calculated by comparing the number of dead animals to those that started the study. The feed supplied and rejected for a period of 24 h was used to calculate the daily feed intake (FI). The initial body weight (BW), final body weight, and the experimental days were used to determine the average daily gain (ADG). Likewise, the feed conversion ratio (FCR) was recorded as the kg of feed consumed to gain 1 kg of BW.

## 2.4. Intestinal Integrity

At 95 days old, 10 rabbits were randomly selected for each treatment. An electrical stun was performed with two electrodes under the following specifications: electricity 125 V, power 160 mA, 0.3 amps, frequency 50 Hz, and duration 2–3 s. After unconsciousness was verified, they were slaughtered, and six samples of intestinal tissue were taken [21].

After the tissues were washed, representative sections (1 cm$^2$ samples) were taken from the middle longitudinal part of the duodenum (the area that corresponds to the junction with the stomach and up to the first intestinal loop) and from the middle longitudinal part of the cecum. Note that one section per intestinal segment (duodenum and cecum) was evaluated. Next, they were placed in 10% formalin in phosphate-buffered saline (pH 7.4) at 4 °C, which was subjected to the histological technique [8], dehydrated in a graduated series of ethanol, and embedded in paraffin. Subsequently, thick samples of 4 to 5 microns were taken with a longitudinal orientation to ensure that the complete layers of the intestine were present.

Next, in the tissues, a routine of deparaffinization, hydration, and staining (hematoxylin-eosin) was followed. Five slides per animal were evaluated, with five serial cuts per slide and five random fields per slide. The thickness of the muscular and mucosal layers in the duodenum and cecum was calculated. Furthermore, in the duodenum, the height, width, and number of villi were quantified. In the cecum, the depth, thickness, and number of the crypts were determined. An Axiostar microscope (Carl Zeiss, Oberkochen, Germany) was connected to a computer with Opti-AnalySIS Basic software, and 500× and 100× images were used to determine all study measurements. Finally, the ratio of villus height/depth of the crypt was calculated [8].

## 2.5. Statistical Analysis

The experimental study considered a completely randomized design. To determine the data normality and the variance uniformity, the Kolmogorov–Smirnov and Bartlett tests were used. Next, the data were processed by a simple classification analysis of variance (ANOVA). Where necessary, a post hoc analysis (Duncan) was used. Likewise, the Kruskal–Wallis test was performed to determine the number of villi and crypts. All analyzes were performed according to the statistical software SPSS version 23.0.

## 3. Results

Table 2 shows that the dietary use of the *Agave tequilana* stem powder did not statistically change the viability and FCR ($p > 0.05$); however, T3 increased BW, FI, and the ADG compared to a basal diet (T0), T1, and T2 during the 60 experimental days ($p < 0.05$).

**Table 2.** Effect of *A. tequilana* stem powder on performance of rabbits (35–95 days old).

| | Treatments | | | | | |
|---|---|---|---|---|---|---|
| Items | T0 | T1 | T2 | T3 | SEM± | *p*-Value |
| Viability (%) | 95.00 | 95.00 | 95.00 | 95.00 | | |
| Initial body weight | 774.89 | 767.75 | 768.5 | 771.66 | 4.430 | 0.890 |
| Final body weight (g) | 2478.89 [b] | 2472.35 [b] | 2468.90 [b] | 2550.06 [a] | 14.728 | 0.041 |
| Feed intake (g/rabbit/day) | 120.49 [b] | 119.60 [b] | 119.50 [b] | 124.81 [a] | 0.437 | <0.001 |
| Average daily gain (g/rabbit/day) | 28.40 [b] | 28.41 [b] | 28.34 [b] | 29.64 [a] | 0.296 | 0.049 |
| Feed conversion ratio | 4.24 | 4.21 | 4.22 | 4.21 | 0.034 | 0.059 |

[a,b] Means with different letters in the same row differ at $p < 0.05$. T0: basal diet; T1: 0.5% of *Agave tequilana* stem powder. T2: 1.0% of *Agave tequilana* stem powder. T3: 1.5% of *Agave tequilana* stem powder.

Changes in the intestinal integrity of rabbits (95 days old) when using increasing levels of *A. tequilana* stem powder are shown in Table 3. T3 significantly ($p < 0.05$) enhanced the thickness of the muscular and mucous layers in the duodenum and cecum. Similar results were found for the height and villi thickness in the duodenum compared to T0, T1, and T2 ($p < 0.05$). However, these last treatments (T0–T2) showed ($p < 0.05$) the highest values for the depth zone of the crypts, without differences ($p > 0.05$) for the crypts thickness in the duodenum. Furthermore, T3 decreased ($p < 0.05$) the depth and crypts thickness in the cecum significantly in relation to the other treatments.

Table 3. Effect of *A. tequilana* stem powder on intestinal integrity of rabbits (95 days old).

| Morphometry (μm) | Treatment | | | | SEM± | p-Value |
|---|---|---|---|---|---|---|
| | T0 | T1 | T2 | T3 | | |
| Duodenum | | | | | | |
| Muscle thickness | 119.20 [b] | 121.72 [b] | 119.88 [b] | 150.00 [a] | 6.786 | <0.001 |
| Mucous thickness | 1063.24 [b] | 1056.56 [b] | 1023.84 [b] | 1199.9 [a] | 31.800 | <0.001 |
| Villi height | 891.70 [b] | 894.12 [b] | 892.22 [b] | 1027.96 [a] | 25.041 | <0.001 |
| Villi thickness | 109.00 [b] | 108.03 [b] | 110.52 [b] | 149.80 [a] | 6.500 | <0.001 |
| Crypt area | 321.21 [a] | 322.15 [a] | 322.24 [a] | 267.32 [b] | 7.589 | <0.001 |
| Crypt depth | 99.55 [a] | 98.65 [a] | 98.20 [a] | 72.68 [b] | 7.215 | <0.001 |
| Crypt thickness | 66.89 | 65.76 | 65.77 | 65.76 | 4.122 | 0.314 |
| Villi/Crypts * | 8.95 [b] | 9.06 [b] | 9.06 [b] | 14.14 [a] | 1.251 | <0.001 |
| Cecum | | | | | | |
| Muscle thickness | 286.79 [b] | 284.00 [b] | 287.32 [b] | 396.04 [a] | 28.069 | <0.001 |
| Mucosa thickness | 425.99 [b] | 426.50 [b] | 428.20 [b] | 441.00 [a] | 3.482 | <0.001 |
| Crypt depth | 244.30 [a] | 243.26 [a] | 245.76 [a] | 228.76 [b] | 4.923 | <0.001 |
| Crypt thickness | 121.36 [a] | 121.28 [a] | 121.75 [a] | 97.84 [b] | 5.730 | <0.001 |

[a,b] Means with different letters in the same row differ at $p < 0.05$. * Villus height/crypt depth. T0: basal diet; T1: 0.5% of *Agave tequilana* stem powder. T2: 1.0% of *Agave tequilana* stem powder. T3: 1.5% of *Agave tequilana* stem powder.

Figure 1 shows that T3 increased ($p < 0.05$) the villi number in the duodenum, although without notable differences among treatments ($p > 0.05$) for the crypts number in both intestinal portions (duodenum and cecum).

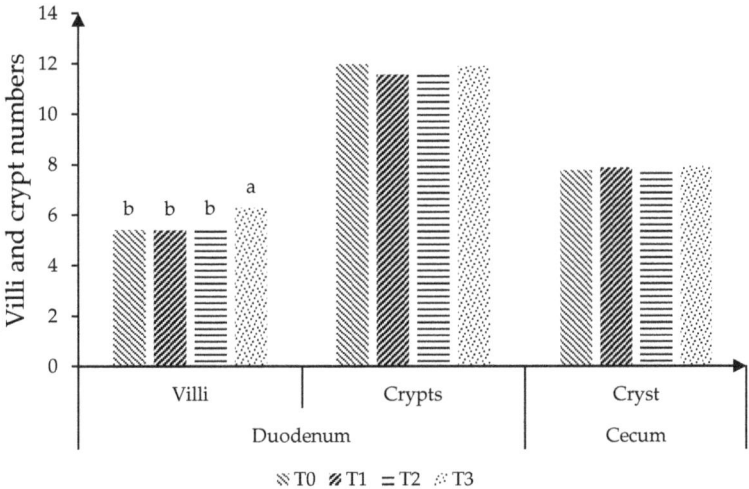

Figure 1. Effect of *A. tequilana* stem powder on the number of villi (SEM ± 0.132; p-value 0.001) and crypts in the duodenum (SEM ± 0.494; p-value 0.088) and on the crypts number (SEM ± 0.259; p-value 0.664) in the cecum of rabbits. [a,b] Means with different letters among treatments differ at $p < 0.05$.

## 4. Discussion

The fact that supplementation of up to 1.5% of *Agave tequilana* stem powder did not change the viability of rabbits (Table 2) confirms that this natural product does not have toxic elements and/or harmful secondary metabolites. Similar results in mortality (6.25%) were found by Iser et al. [8] and Iser et al. [16] when they used up to 1.5% of *A. tequilana* and *A. fourcroydes* stem powder as a natural growth promoter. Likewise, Chávez et al. [14] and Sánchez et al. [15] informed us about a high viability in poultry and pigs when they carried out dietary experiments with dried-stem powder or *Agave tequilana* extract, thus demonstrating the safety of the tested natural product.

On the other hand, in laboratory animals, *Agave tequilana* fructans have been found to modulate the intestinal microbiota, the immune response, the anti-inflammatory activity, and the circulation of harmful serum lipids, which causes a maintenance of or reduction in body weight [22,23]. However, in the case of using rabbits as laboratory animals, T3 increased their body weight by 2.87% and their ADG by 4.37% when compared to the control group (Table 2). The growth-promoting effect of these products rich in fructans will apparently depend on the amount of this carbohydrate in the diet and the category and species of the animal under experimentation. Moreover, Santos-Zea et al. [24] have informed us that the *Agave tequila* stem is rich in secondary metabolites such as polyphenols and saponins, which are considered anti-nutritional factors. However, in adequate concentrations, these chemical compounds have antioxidant and anti-inflammatory effects that decrease low density lipoprotein (LDL) oxidation and regulate cell growth [25]. Apparently, the combined effect of fructans and the beneficial secondary metabolites had a positive effect on rabbits, although more experiments are necessary to verify this approach.

Table 2 also demonstrates that dietary use with dried-stem powder of *A. tequilana* (T3) provoked a higher feed intake (3.59%) and no change in feed conversion, which promoted a higher body weight, suggesting that perhaps favorable conditions in the gastrointestinal tract (GIT) demanded a higher intake of nutrients and energy (Table 3). Previous studies with agave stem (*tequilana* and *fourcroydes*) reported a higher feed intake associated with an increased weight gain in rabbits [8,16]. *Agave tequilana* stem powder also promoted feed intake due to the moderately sweet taste of this natural product as a result of the high concentration of fructans and fructose [26]. Furthermore, other studies using prebiotic compounds in rabbits are contradictory; Mourão et al. [27] and Bovera et al. [28] found that the dietary use with mannanoligosaccharides as a growth-promoter in rabbits increased feed intake, but Alvarado-Loza et al. [29] reported lower intake when they used insulin as part of the rabbit diet. The results (Table 2) demonstrate that dietary supplementation up to 1.5% of *Agave tequilana* stem powder has a natural growth-promoting effect in rabbits. This was supported by other research using *Agave fourcroydes* dried-stem as a prebiotic additive in broiler rabbits [8].

Additionally, *Agave tequilana* stem supplementation (1.5%) changed the thickness of the muscular and mucous layers in broiler rabbits; these intestinal layers are the most significant in digestive morphophysiology and in the diagnosis of digestive diseases; the first contributes to peristalsis and the movement of the feed chyme, which directs it along and out of the intestines, and the second produces mucus, lubricates the passage of the food chyme, and protects the GIT from the action of digestive enzymes [30]. Thus, an increase in the thickness of these intestinal layers (muscle and mucosa) with T3 is associated with higher intestinal health [6]. These results may be associated with a decrease in intestinal pH due to the increase in the population of cecal lactic acid bacteria (BAL), already confirmed by Martínez et al. [31] when using *Agave fourcroydes* stem powder (with similar chemical characteristics to *Agave tequilana*) up to 1.5% in rabbit diets. In this sense, Revolledo et al. [32] have informed us that better intestinal health, due to decreased adherence of pathogenic bacteria and intestinal damage due to competitive exclusion of bacteria, has a direct effect on the concentric layers thickness.

Furthermore, de Blas et al. [33] found a reduction in the thickness of the mucous layer due to the greater presence of *Helicobacter* spp., *Campylobacter* spp. and *C. perfringens*, which increased the mortality and decreased the productive response of rabbits. This intestinal layer is related to tissues involved in the defense of the host against infectious diseases. This allows for better immune activity and modulation of the intestinal barrier [32], which directly affect the productive performance of animals [3].

On the other hand, Raj et al. [34] reported that there is a close relationship between the thickness of the intestinal mucosa and the intestinal barrier. These authors reported that a significant decrease in this intestinal layer can decrease intestinal permeability due to the unlimited access of toxins, microorganisms, substances, macromolecules, and chemicals, which could cause gastrointestinal disturbances that directly affect animal productivity. It should be noted that the mucous layer thickness is greater in the duodenum than in the cecum due to absorptive activity in this portion. However, the muscle layer thickness is more significant due to the transport of feces, especially in rabbits due to cecotrophy [20].

Additionally, some authors [35] have suggested that the histo-morphometry of the villi and crypts are directly related to intestinal health and animal response. Thus, these results showed that the better conditions of the intestinal environment, due to a higher proliferation of lactic acid bacteria (LAB) [31] provided by T3, led to an increase ($p < 0.05$) in the height and thickness of the villi, and in the thickness of the intestinal mucosa (Table 3), thus denoting a more developed intestinal tissue. Other experiments with productive animals using high-fructan diets have reported similar responses in villus height and width [30,31]. The authors associated these results with greater health and intestinal absorption area. However, the studies by Mourão et al. [27], when they used diets with fructooligosaccharides in rabbits, did not find notable changes ($p > 0.05$) for these indicators.

It has been verified that the use of nutraceutical foods intervenes in the development of the GIT, especially in "villi height and crypts depth," as well as in productive efficiency, nutrient absorption capacity, and reduction of metabolic requirements [35]. In this sense, the relationship of the villi height/crypts depth is used as a nutritional and health indicator to estimate the digestive processes and the absorption of nutrients in the gut [36]. Thus, the greatest capacity for digestion and absorption occurs when this ratio increases [37,38]. According to Vallejos et al. [30], a shortening of the intestinal villi in relation to a greater depth of the crypt causes a decrease in absorption cells and more secretory cells. On the other hand, the highest supplementation with *Agave tequilana* stem powder (1.5%) decreased the thickness and depth of the crypts in the duodenum (Table 3). According to Cai et al. [6], in apparently healthy animals, a greater crypt depth is related to the migration of specialized cells towards the villi, influenced by the shortening and decreased functionality of these structures due to multifactorial causes, although with greater emphasis due to the microbial dysbiosis. Likewise, other studies on the dietary use of up to 1.5% *Agave fourcroydes* stem powder compared to the control treatment showed a higher ratio of these intestinal structures [8]. It is noteworthy that the intestine has a rapid epithelial renewal, due to the shortening of the deep Lieberkühn crypts [33].

At the same time, in previous research, Iser et al. [8] reported that the dietary use of *Agave fourcroydes* stem powder (up to 1.5%) enhanced the number of intestinal villi, due to better gut health, which promoted the growth of rabbits. To our knowledge, this is the first study showing the effect of *Agave tequilana* powder on intestinal histo-morphometry of rabbits. Moreover, the number and size of the villi will depend on the number of cells that compose it. In this way, the functional integrity of the villi cells, both in the luminal membrane and in the base-lateral membrane, are directly related to the absorption of nutrients [39]. It is important to clarify that each villus corresponds to a crypt; the numerical difference in the duodenum is due to the cross section made to the tissues for this analysis [30].

Generally, gastrointestinal problems in human beings and animals provoke changes in the villi structure (mainly atrophy or shortening), especially due to the presence of pathogenic bacteria or other associated pathologies [38]. As mentioned above, in these apparently healthy animals (rabbits), supplementation with *Agave tequilana* powder (1.5%) increased the villi thickness and decreased the crypts depth, which provoked a reduction in the inter-villus space, with a greater quantification of these filaments (villi) at a field reading with 100× and 500× under the microscope. In this sense, Gālina et al. [40] found that various nutraceuticals increased the number of intestinal villi in an apparently healthy animal model. In a similar vein, Mourao et al. [28] suggested that the diets with mannan-oligosaccharides provoked a greater height of intestinal villi, associated with the growth of beneficial cecal bacteria in rabbits. This shows that the number of functional villi in the duodenum changes due to the effect of the diet supplied, considering that dietary treatments did not cause enteric problems in these rabbits.

## 5. Conclusions

The results indicate that the dietary supplementation of 1.5% of *A. tequilana* (Weber var. Azul) stem powder in broiler rabbits (35–95 days old) improved the growth performance and histomorphometry of the concentric layers (muscle and mucosa), villi, and crypts as indicators of intestinal health, which justified the natural growth-promoting effect of this product in rabbit production.

**Author Contributions:** Conceptualization, Y.M., M.R., D.S. and M.I.; methodology Y.M., D.S., M.I., M.R. and E.A.; software, Y.M., M.I., M.R. and E.A.; validation, Y.M., M.I., M.R. and E.A.; formal analysis, Y.M. and M.I., investigation, Y.M., D.S., M.R., M.I. and M.V.; resources, D.S., M.R. and E.A.; data curation, M.R. and E.A.; writing—original draft preparation, Y.M. and M.I.; writing—review and editing, Y.M., M.I. and M.V.; visualization, Y.M.; supervision, Y.M., M.R. and D.S.; project administration, Y.M., M.R. and D.S.; funding acquisition, Y.M., M.R., D.S. and E.A. All authors have read and agreed to the published version of the manuscript.

**Funding:** This research received no external funding.

**Institutional Review Board Statement:** The Veterinary Medicine Division of the University Center for Biological and Agricultural Sciences of the Guadalajara University, Jalisco, Mexico, reviewed and approved all the standardized procedures performed in this experiment, which was carried out under the Mexican animal welfare guidelines and the experimental and "NORMA Oficial Mexicana NOM-033-SAG/ZOO-2014, Methods for slaughter domestic and wild animals (Reference number: CINV. 106/12).

**Informed Consent Statement:** Not applicable.

**Data Availability Statement:** The data presented in this study are available on request from the corresponding author.

**Conflicts of Interest:** The authors declare no conflict of interest.

## References

1. Allen, H.K. Antibiotic resistance gene discovery in food-producing animals. *Curr. Opin. Microbiol.* **2014**, *19*, 25–29. [CrossRef] [PubMed]
2. Ayed, H.; Saïd, B. Effect of Tiamulin or Rescue-kit® on diet utilisation, growth and carcass yield of growing rabbits. *World Rabbit. Sci.* **2008**, *16*, 183–188. [CrossRef]
3. Liu, G.; Aguilar, Y.M.; Zhang, L.; Ren, W.; Chen, S.; Guan, G.; Xiong, X.; Liao, P.; Li, T.; Huang, R.; et al. Dietary supplementation with sanguinarine enhances serum metabolites and antibodies in growing pigs. *J. Anim. Sci.* **2016**, *94*, 75–78. [CrossRef]
4. Colitti, M.; Stefanon, B.; Gabai, G.; Gelain, M.E.; Bonsembiante, F. Oxidative stress and nutraceuticals in the modulation of the immune function: Current knowledge in animals of veterinary interest. *Antioxidants* **2019**, *8*, 28. [CrossRef]
5. Sun, H.; Ni, X.; Song, X.; Wen, B.; Zhou, Y.; Zou, F.; Yang, M.; Peng, Z.; Zhu, H.; Zeng, Y.; et al. Fermented Yupingfeng polysaccharides enhance immunity by improving the foregut microflora and intestinal barrier in weaning rex rabbits. *Appl. Microbiol. Biotechnol.* **2016**, *100*, 8105–8120. [CrossRef] [PubMed]
6. Cai, Y.; Aguilar, Y.; Yu, L.; Wan, Y.; Liu, H.; Liu, G.; Zhong, J.; Jiang, Y.B.; Yin, Y.L. Effects of dietary supplementation of *Lactobacillus plantarum* on growth performance and serum concentration of amino acids in weaned piglets. *Anim. Nutr. Feed Technol.* **2014**, *14*, 411–420. [CrossRef]
7. Liu, G.; Yu, L.; Martínez, Y.; Ren, W.; Ni, H.; Abdullah Al-Dhabi, N.; Duraipandiyan, V.; Yin, Y. Dietary Saccharomyces cerevisiae cell wall extract supplementation alleviates oxidative stress and modulates serum amino acids profiles in weaned piglets. *Oxid. Med. Cell Longev.* **2017**, *2017*, 3967439. [CrossRef]
8. Iser, M.; Martinez, Y.; Ni, H.; Jiang, H.; Valdivie Navarro, M.; Wu, X.; Al-Dhabi, N.A.; Rosales, M.; Duraipandiyan, V.; Fang, J. Effects of *Agave fourcroydes* powder as a dietary supplement on growth performance, gut morphology, concentration of IgG and hematology parameters of broiler rabbits. *Biomed Res. Int.* **2016**, *2016*, 3414319. [CrossRef]

9. Shen, X.; Cui, H.; Xu, X. Orally administered *Lactobacillus casei* exhibited several probiotic properties in artificially suckling rabbits. *Asian Australas. J. Anim. Sci.* **2020**, *33*, 1352–1359. [CrossRef]
10. Gust, G. ¡Tequila! A natural and cultural history. *Econ. Botany* **2004**, *58*, 750. [CrossRef]
11. García, Y.; Ayala, L.; Bocourt, R.; Albelo, N.; Nuñez, O.; Rodríguez, Y.; López, M.G. Agavins as prebiotic. Their influence on lipid metabolism of pigs. *Cuban J. Agric. Sci.* **2018**, *52*, 395–400. Available online: http://scielo.sld.cu/scielo.php?script=sci_abstract&pid=S2079-34802018000400395&lng=es&nrm=iso&tlng=en (accessed on 10 February 2021).
12. López, G.; Mancilla, M.; Mendoza, D. Molecular structures of fructans from *Agave tequilana* Weber azul. *J. Agric. Food Chem.* **2003**, *51*, 7835–7840. [CrossRef] [PubMed]
13. Salazar-Leyva, J.A.; Osuna-Ruiz, I.; Rodríguez-Tirado, V.A.; Zazueta-Patrón, I.E.; Brito-Rojas, H.D. Optimization study of fructans extraction from *Agave tequilana* Weber azul variety. *Food Sci. Technol.* **2016**, *36*, 631–637. [CrossRef]
14. Chavez-Mora, I.; Sanchez-Chipres, D.; Galindo-García, J.; Ayala-Valdovinos, M.A.; Duifhuis-Rivera, T.; Ly, J. Efecto de oligofructosa de agave en dietas de gallinas ponedoras en la producción de huevos. *Rev. MVZ Córdoba* **2019**, *24*, 7108–7112. [CrossRef]
15. Sanchez-Chiprés, D.S.; Leal, E.; Galindo, J.; Valdovinos, M.A.; Ly, J. Features of carcass performance and characteristics and meat quality in pigs fed agave oligofructans. *Cuban J. Agric. Sci.* **2018**, *52*, 41–48. Available online: http://scielo.sld.cu/pdf/cjas/v52n1/2079-3480-cjas-52-01-41.pdf (accessed on 15 December 2021).
16. Iser, M.; Martínez, Y.; Valdivié, M.; Sánchez, D.; Rosales, M. Comportamiento productivo y características de la canal de conejos alimentados con harina de *Agave tequilana*. *Rev. Electrón. Vet.* **2016**, *17*, 1–12. Available online: https://www.redalyc.org/pdf/636/63647454008.pdf (accessed on 15 December 2021).
17. Iser, M.; Valdivié, M.; Sánchez, D.; Rosales, M.; Más, D.; Martínez, Y. Effect of dietary supplementation with *Agave tequilana* stems powder on hematological and blood biochemical indicators of rabbits. *Cuban J. Agric. Sci.* **2019**, *53*, 1–7. Available online: http://scielo.sld.cu/scielo.php?script=sci_arttext&pid=S2079-34802019000400403 (accessed on 15 December 2021).
18. AOAC. *Official Methods of Analysis of AOAC*, 18th ed.; Association of Official Analytical Chemists: Gaithersburg, MD, USA, 2006.
19. Van Soest, P.; Robertson, J.; Lewis, B. Methods for dietary fiber, neutral detergent fiber, and non-starch polysaccharides in relation to animal nutrition. *J. Dairy Sci.* **1991**, *74*, 3583–3597. [CrossRef]
20. de Blas, J.; Mateos, G. Feed formulation. In *The Nutrition of the Rabbit*, 2nd ed.; De Blas, C., Wiseman, J., Eds.; CABI Publishing: Oxon, UK; CAB International: Wallingford, UK, 2010; pp. 222–232.
21. Norma Oficial Mexicana. *Métodos para dar Muerte a los Animales Domésticos y Silvestres*; NOM-033-SAG/ZOO; SAGARPA: Ciudad de Mexico, Mexico, 2014; pp. 21–23. Available online: https://www.gob.mx/cms/uploads/attachment/file/133499/4.-_NORMA_OFICIAL_MEXICANA_NOM-033-SAG-ZOO-2014.pdf (accessed on 15 November 2021).
22. Márquez-Aguirre, A.L.; Camacho-Ruiz, R.M.; Arriaga-Alba, M.; Padilla-Camberos, E.; Kirchmayr, M.R.; Blasco, J.L.; González-Avila, M. Effects of *Agave tequilana* fructans with different degree of polymerization profiles on the body weight, blood lipids and count of fecal Lactobacilli/Bifidobacteria in obese mice. *Food Funct.* **2013**, *4*, 1237–1244. [CrossRef]
23. Padilla-Camberos, E.; Barragán-Álvarez, C.P.; Diaz-Martinez, N.E.; Rathod, V.; Flores-Fernández, J.M. Effects of Agave fructans (*Agave tequilana* Weber var. azul) on body fat and serum lipids in obesity. *Plant. Food Hum. Nutr.* **2018**, *73*, 34–39. [CrossRef]
24. Santos-Zea, L.; Leal-Diaz, A.; Cortes-Ceballos, E.; Gutierrez-Uribe, J. Agave (*Agave* spp.) and its traditional products as a source of bioactive compounds. *Curr. Bioact. Compd.* **2012**, *8*, 218–231. [CrossRef]
25. Tlili, N.; Sarikurkcu, C. Bioactive compounds profile, enzyme inhibitory and antioxidant activities of water extract from five selected medicinal plants. *Ind. Crop. Product.* **2020**, *151*, 112448. [CrossRef]
26. Mellado-Mojica, E.; López-Pérez, M.G. Comparative analysis between blue agave syrup (*Agave tequilana* Weber var. azul) and other natural syrups. *Agrociencia* **2013**, *47*, 233–244. Available online: http://www.scielo.org.mx/scielo.php?pid=S1405-31952013000300003&script=sci_abstract&tlng=en (accessed on 15 December 2021).
27. Mourão, J.; Pinheiro, V.; Alves, A.; Guedes, C.; Pinto, L.; Saavedra, M.; Spring, P.; Kocher, A. Effect of mannan oligosaccharides on the performance, intestinal morphology and cecal fermentation in rabbits. *Anim. Feed Sci. Technol.* **2006**, *126*, 107–120. [CrossRef]
28. Bovera, F.; Marono, S.; Nizza, S.; Mallardo, M.; Grossi, M.; Piccolo, V. Use of mannan oligosaccharides during post-weaning enteric syndrome in rabbits: Effect on in vivo performance from 35 to 60 days. *Ital. J. Anim. Sci.* **2009**, *8*, 775–777. [CrossRef]
29. Alvarado-Loza, E.; Orozco-Hernández, R.; Ruíz-García, I.; Paredes-Ibarra, F.; Fuentes-Hernández, V. The 2% of agave inulin level in the rabbit feed affects positively the digestibility and gut microbia. *Abanico Vet.* **2017**, *7*, 55–62.
30. Vallejos, D.; Carcelén, F.; Jiménez, R.; Perales, R.; Santillán, G.; Ara, M.; Carzola, F. Effect of sodium butyrate supplementation on fattening guinea pig (*Cavia porcellus*) diets on the development of intestinal villi and crypts of Lieberkühn. *Rev. Investig. Vet. Perú.* **2015**, *26*, 395–403.
31. Martínez, Y.; Iser, M.; Valdivié, M.; Galindo, J.; Sánchéz, D. Supplementation with *Agave fourcroydes* powder on growth performance, carcass traits, organ weights, gut morphometry, and blood biochemistry in broiler rabbits. *Rev. Mex. Cienc. Pecu.* **2021**, *12*, 756–772. [CrossRef]
32. Revolledo, L.; Ferreira, J.; Mead, G. Prospects in Salmonella control: Competitive exclusion, probiotics, and enhancement of avian intestinal immunity. *J. Appl. Poultry. Res.* **2006**, *15*, 341–351. [CrossRef]
33. De Blas, J.C.; Chamorro, S.; García-Alonso, J.; García-Rebollar, P.; García-Ruiz, A.I.; Gómez-Conde, M.S.; Menoyo, D.; Nicodemus, N.; Romero, C.; Carabaño, R. Nutritional digestive disturbances in weaner rabbits. *Anim. Feed Sci. Technol.* **2012**, *173*, 102–110. [CrossRef]

34. Raj, A.S.; Holtmann, G.; Fletcher, L.; Vesey, D.A.; Hickman, I.J.; Shanahan, E.R.; Tran, C.D.; Macdonald, G. Altered proximal small-intestinal permeability and bacterial translocation in chronic liver disease in relation to hepatic fibrosis and disease severity. *Gastroenterology* **2016**, *12*, 1729–17448. [CrossRef]
35. Jiang, J.F.; Song, X.M.; Huang, X.; Zhou, W.D.; Wu, J.L.; Zhu, Z.G.; Zheng, H.C.; Jiang, Y.Q. Effects of alfalfa powder on growth performance and gastrointestinal tract development of growing ducks. *Asian Austral. J. Anim. Sci.* **2012**, *25*, 1445–1450. [CrossRef] [PubMed]
36. Pinheiro, V.; Guedes, C.; Outor, D.; Mourao, J. Effects of fibre level and dietary man-nanoligosacharides on digestibility, caecal volatile fatty acids and performances of growing rabbits. *Anim. Feed Sci. Technol.* **2009**, *148*, 288–300. [CrossRef]
37. Pérez, C.; Vasco, B.; Colina, I.; Machado, I.; Rossini, M.; Arrieta, D. Effect of the addition of enzyme complexes in sorghum (*Sorghum bicolor*) based diets on intestinal integrity of broilers. *Rev. Cient. Fac. Cien. Vet.* **2013**, *23*, 59–66. Available online: https://produccioncientificaluz.org/index.php/cientifica/article/view/15776 (accessed on 10 November 2021).
38. Montagne, L.; Boudry, G.; Favier, C.; Huërou, C.; Lallès, P.; Seve, B. Main intestinal markers associated with the changes in gut architecture and function in piglets after weaning. *Brit. J. Nutr.* **2007**, *97*, 45–57. [CrossRef] [PubMed]
39. Patra, A.K.; Amasheh, S.; Aschenbach, J.R. Modulation of gastrointestinal barrier and nutrient transport function in farm animals by natural plant bioactive compounds–A comprehensive review. *Crit. Rev. Food Sci. Nutr.* **2019**, *59*, 3237–3266. [CrossRef]
40. Gāliņa, D.; Ansonska, L.; Valdovska, A. Effect of Probiotics and herbal products on intestinal histomorphological and immunological development in piglets. *Vet. Med. Int.* **2020**, *2020*, 3461768. [CrossRef] [PubMed]

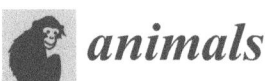

Article

# Preventive Potential of Dipeptide Enterocin A/P on Rabbit Health and Its Effect on Growth, Microbiota, and Immune Response

Monika Pogány Simonová [1,*], Ľubica Chrastinová [2], Jana Ščerbová [1], Valentína Focková [1], Iveta Plachá [1], Zuzana Formelová [2], Mária Chrenková [2] and Andrea Lauková [1]

[1] Centre of Biosciences of the Slovak Academy of Sciences, Institute of Animal Physiology, Šoltésovej 4-6, 040 01 Kosice, Slovakia; scerbova@saske.sk (J.Š.); fockova@saske.sk (V.F.); placha@saske.sk (I.P.); laukova@saske.sk (A.L.)
[2] National Agricultural and Food Centre, Hlohovecká 2, 951 41 Lužianky, Slovakia; lubica.chrastinova@nppc.sk (Ľ.C.); zuzana.formelova@nppc.sk (Z.F.); maria.chrenkova@nppc.sk (M.C.)
* Correspondence: simonova@saske.sk; Tel.: +421-55-7922964

**Simple Summary:** Rabbits are animals sensitive to alimentary disturbances and various spoilage agents, mostly during the weaning period. For this reason, the use of natural feed additives has become an area of research in rabbit nutrition, mainly with a focus on prevention. The "in vivo" administration of bacteriocins/enterocins shows an increasing potential in the prevention/treatment of animals' diseases. Therefore, our study focused on the preventive potential of the dipeptide enterocin (Ent) A/P against the methicillin-resistant (MR) *Staphylococcus epidermidis* SE P3/Tr2a strain in rabbit model, determining its effect on the growth performance, phagocytic activity, secretory (s) IgA, and gut microbial composition of rabbits. Ent A/P increased the weight gain of rabbits and its antibacterial effect showed a tendency to stabilize and improve gut microbiota due to reduction of MR staphylococci, total bacteria, and coliforms. The immune-stimulatory effect of Ent A/P was noted due to increased phagocytic activity. Achieved results showed the great potential of Ent A/P application as a feed additive in rabbit nutrition to improve the health and productivity of animals.

**Abstract:** The present study investigated the effect of the dipeptide enterocin (Ent) A/P on growth, immune response, and intestinal microbiota in rabbits. Eighty-eight rabbits (aged five weeks, M91 meat line, both sexes) were divided into three experimental groups: E (Ent A/P; 50 µL/animal/day for 14 days; between 0–14 days); S (methicillin-resistant *Staphylococcus epidermidis* SE P3/Tr2a strain; 500 µL/animal/day for 7 days starting at day 14 to day 21); and E + S (Ent A/P between 0–14 days and SE P3/Tr2a strain between 14–21 days) groups, and the control group (C). The additives were administered in drinking water. Administration of Ent A/P lead to an increase in weight gain, reduction of feed conversion; phagocytic activity was stimulated and gut microbiota were optimized due to reduction of coliforms, total bacterial count, and methicillin-resistant staphylococci. Good health and increased weight gain also showed that methicillin-resistant *S. epidermidis* SE P3/Tr2a strain did not have any pathogenic effect on rabbits' health status.

**Keywords:** enterocin; rabbit; health; immunity; microbiota; prevention

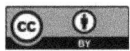

## 1. Introduction

The routine and indiscriminate use of conventional antibiotics in agriculture presents a growing threat, leading to an increase in drug-resistant bacteria in animals and their transmission to humans. Current research is focusing on alternative antimicrobial compounds for use in animal production and veterinary medicine. Bacteriocins are antimicrobial proteins with a broad antibacterial spectrum produced by Gram-positive and Gram-negative bacteria, mostly by lactic acid bacteria (LAB), including enterococci (producing bacteriocins named mostly enterocins; [1]), currently indicated for use in food preservation, but they also have great potential in the prevention and treatment of animals' diseases. Bacteriocins/enterocins have a low tendency to develop resistance compared to conventional antibiotics and they are characterized by biosafety and several bioactive roles–they possess antimicrobial, anticancer, antioxidant, and immunomodulatory effects [2–5]. Therefore, bacteriocins could be a promising alternative as feed additives in livestock farms to improve the health and productivity of food animals. Regarding their success to eliminate multi-drug resistant (MDR) bacteria, they can also be applied in several areas of veterinary medicine with preventive effects and/or to treat bacterial infections [4,6,7].

MDR bacteria represent a public health problem worldwide, with the focus mainly on vancomycin-resistant enterococci, carbapenem-resistant enterobacteria, and pseudomonads. There is also a focus on methicillin-resistant *Staphylococcus aureus* (MRSA) and other coagulase-positive (MRCoPS) and coagulase-negative staphylococci (MRCoNS) [8]. While MRSA in human medicine is detected mostly as hospital-acquired MRSA (HA-MRSA), in veterinary medicine methicillin-resistant staphylococci (MRS) are causative agents of cows' mastitis, chickens' lameness, pigs' exudative epidermitis, canine pyoderma, skin lesions in dogs and cats, and abscesses, mastitis, and septicemia in rabbits [9,10]. Because of a great diversity of MRS host species–pets, food, and wild animals [11]–a special attention is required regarding MRS' co-resistance to other antibiotics, influencing the antimicrobial therapeutic effect and offering a source of resistance genes for other staphylococcal species. For this reason, new antimicrobial agents directed against antibiotic-resistant bacteria, such as bacteriocins, are requested. In vitro bacteriocins testing against MRS, MRSA, and multi-drug resistant staphylococci (MDRS) showed promising results, including their antimicrobial and antibiofilm effect [12–14], confirmed also in several animal models, mostly in the murine model [3]. While the anti-MRSA resp. anti-MRS activity of bacteriocins was presented in a number of papers, mostly during lantibiotics' testing, the effect of enterocins on MRS isolates are documented only in some studies [15–17]. Moreover, most of the mentioned in vivo experiments present the therapeutic effect of bacteriocins tested in animal models [3], but the prevention of pathogenic and resistant bacteria multiplication using bacteriocins as feed additives is also important.

Therefore, the aim of this study was to test the preventive effect of a dipeptide enterocin (Ent) A/P (previously named Ent EK13, produced by *Enterococcus faecium* EK13 strain deponed to the Czech Collection of Microorganisms in Brno, Czech Republic with no. CCM7419 [18]) against methicillin-resistant *Staphylococcus epidermidis* SE P3/Tr2a strain in a rabbit model. The effect on growth performance, immune response, *Eimeria* spp. oocysts' occurrence, and the intestinal microbiota composition of rabbits was controlled.

## 2. Materials and Methods

### 2.1. Animals Care and Use

The experiment was performed in cooperation with our colleagues at the experimental rabbit facility of the National Agricultural and Food Centre, Research Institute for Animal Production, Nitra, Slovakia. All applicable international, national and/or institutional guidelines for the care and use of animals were followed appropriately, and all experimental procedures were approved by the Institutional Ethic Committee (permission code: SK CH 17016 and SK U 18016) and the State Veterinary and Food Administration of the Slovak Republic (4047/16-221).

### 2.2. Experiment Schedule, and Diet

A total of 88 post-weaned hybrid rabbits, (meat lines M91 and P91, weaned at the age of 35 days, both sexes, equal male to female ratio per treatment), were used in this experiment. Rabbits were divided into three experimental groups (E, S, E + S) and one control group (CG), with 22 animals in each group. The average live weight of rabbits at the start of the experiment was 1091.8 g ± 149.3. The rabbits were kept in standard metal cages (61 × 34 × 33 cm, Kovobel company, Domažlice, Czech Republic), two animals per cage. A cycle of 16 h of light and 8 h of dark was used throughout the experiment. Temperature (20 ± 4 °C) and humidity (70 ± 5%) were maintained throughout the experiment by heating and ventilation systems, and data were recorded continuously with a digital thermograph positioned at the same level as the cages. Animals were fed a commercial pelleted diet for growing rabbits (KV, Tekro-Nitra, Ltd., Nitra, Slovakia; Table 1) during the whole experiment with access to water *ad libitum*. The ingredients and chemical composition of this diet are presented in Table 1. The chemical analyses were conducted according to AOAC [19] and Van Soest et al. [20]. The animals in group E were administered Ent A/P (prepared according to Mareková et al. [21]), a dose of 50 µL/animal/day, with activity of 25,600 AU/mL during the first 14 days of the treatment period (between days 0/1 and 14), to control the preventive effect of tested enterocin A/P (Figure 1). The activity of Ent A/P was tested by the agar spot test according to De Vuyst et al. [22] against the principal indicator strain *E. avium* EA5 (isolated from the feces of piglets, our laboratory). Rabbits in group S received only the methicillin-resistant *Staphylococcus epidermidis* SE P3/Tr2a strain ($1.0 \times 10^5$ CFU/mL; Pogány Simonová et al. [17]) in their drinking water at a dose of 500µL/animal/day for 7 days, between 14 and 21 days. The strain was marked by rifampicin to differentiate it from the total staphylococci and prepared as described previously by Strompfová et al. [23]. Rabbits in the E + S group firstly consumed the Ent A/P for 14 days (between 0–14 days) and after it the SE P3/Tr2a strain was applied to animals for 7 days, starting at day 14 (when the Ent A/P application was ceased), and finishing at day 21 of the trial. Based on our previous experiments, that these additives can be dissolved in distilled water [21], the additives were applied firstly to 100 mL of drinking water in all cages to ensure that rabbits received the applied additives, and after consuming this volume the rabbits had access to water ad libitum. Control rabbits (group C) had the same conditions, but without additives being applied to their drinking water, and they were fed a commercial diet. Drinking water was provided through nipple drinkers. The experiment lasted for 21 days.

**Table 1.** Nutrient content of commercial granulated diet for growing rabbits.

| Nutrient Content | g·kg$^{-1}$ in Original Feed | g·kg$^{-1}$ in Dry Matter |
|---|---|---|
| Dry matter | 886.65 | 1000.00 |
| Crude protein | 155.35 | 174.94 |
| Crude fiber | 132.37 | 149.29 |
| Crude fat | 20.30 | 22.89 |
| Ash | 90.08 | 101.60 |
| Starch | 238.71 | 269.22 |
| Acid detergent fiber | 151.69 | 171.08 |
| Neutral detergent fiber | 295.10 | 332.83 |
| Calcium | 15.90 | 17.94 |
| Phosphorus | 4.89 | 5.51 |
| Magnesium | 2.57 | 2.90 |
| Sodium potassium | 1.21 | 1.36 |
| Iron | 564.70 * | 636.88 * |
| Zinc | 97.77 * | 110.27 * |
| Copper | 20.50 * | 23.12 * |
| Metabolizable energy (MJ.kg−1) | 11.16 | 11.02 |

* mg·kg$^{-1}$ feed.

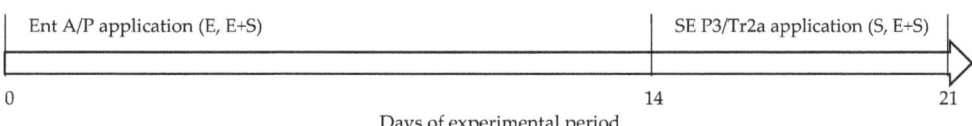

**Figure 1.** Scheme of the Ent A/P and S. epidermidis SE P3/Tr2a strain application.

### 2.3. Growth Performance

Body weight (BW) and feed consumption were measured every week during the experiment; average daily weight gain (ADWG) and feed conversion ratio (FCR) were calculated mathematically. Mortality was recorded daily throughout the whole experiment.

### 2.4. Phagocytic Activity in Blood

For phagocytic activity (PA), blood ($n$ = 8) was sampled from the marginal ear vein (*Vena auricularis*) into Eppendorf tubes containing micro-spheric hydrophilic (MSH) particles and heparin at days 0, 14, and 21. Briefly, 50 µL of MSH particle suspension (ARTIM, Prague, Czech Republic) was mixed with 100 µL of blood in an Eppendorf-type test tube and incubated at 37 °C for 1 h. Blood smears were then prepared and stained in accordance with May–Grünwald and Giemsa–Romanowski, and the direct microscopic counting procedure, calculating the number of white cells containing at least three engulfed particles per 100 white cells (monocytes/granulocytes), was used for PA analysis [24].

### 2.5. Immunoglobulin A in Small Intestinal Wall

Eight rabbits in each group were killed at 21 days of the trial (56 d of age) using electronarcosis (50 Hz, 0.3 A/rabbit for 5 s), immediately hung by the hind legs on the processing line and quickly bled by cutting the jugular veins and the carotid arteries. Samples ($n$ = 8) of the small intestine were collected for IgA analyses, and the appendix and cecum contents for microbial analysis.

The concentration of immunoglobulin A (IgA) in the intestinal wall was measured using the competitive inhibition enzyme immunoassay technique (Rabbit Immunoglobulin A, IgA ELISA kit, Cusabio, Houston, TX, USA). Samples of intestinal wall were prepared according to Nikawa et al. [25] and analyzed using the Multireader Synergy HTX (Biotek, Shoreline, WA, USA), at the wavelength 450 nm according to the manufacturer of Cusabio kit.

### 2.6. Microbial Analyses and Eimeria spp. Oocysts Detection

Freshly-voided feces were collected using nets mounted under the cages, five nets under 11 cages. Because there were two animals housed in each cage, and in some places the feces were mixed, we decided to collect mixed samples, one mixed sample per net, i.e., five mixture samples per group. Feces were sampled at day 0/1 (at the start of the experiment and Ent A/P application; 10 mixture samples from all rabbits, respectively, from all groups together–initial microbial background, at day 14 (2 weeks after the start of the experiment; the end of Ent A/P and the start of the *S. epidermidis* SE P3/Tr2a strain application; five mixture samples from each group) and at day 21 (56 days of age; the end of SE P3/Tr2a strain application). For microbial testing, samples of feces, cecum, and appendix contents (1 g) were treated using the standard microbiological dilution method (International Organization for Standardization (ISO)). The appropriate dilutions in Ringer solution (pH 7.0; Oxoid Ltd., Basingstoke, Hampshire, England) were plated onto the following media: M-Enterococus Agar (NF-V04503, Difco Laboratories, Detroit, MI, USA) for enterococci, M17 Agar (Difco) for streptococci, MacConkey agar (ISO 7402, Oxoid) for coliforms, Mannitol Salt Agar for coagulase-negative staphylococci (CoNS, ISO 6888), Plate Count Agar (Biomark Laboratories, Pune, India) for total bacterial growth, Oxacillin Resistance Screening Agar (Oxoid) to confirm methicillin-resistant staphylococci. Brain-Heart Infusion agar (Difco) enriched with rifampicin (Rifasynt, Medochemie Ltd., Limassol, Cyprus) was used to determine *S. epidermidis* P3/Tr2a. Bacteria were cultivated at 30 °C and/or 37 °C for 24–48 h depending on the bacterial genera and their counts were expressed in log 10 of colony forming units per gram (log 10 CFU/g ± SD). Randomly picked up representatives of selected bacterial groups were confirmed by MALDI-TOF identification system (Bruker Daltonics, Billerica, MA, USA).

Fecal samples were stored at 4 °C and examined for the *Eimeria* spp. oocysts by the flotation technique, according to McMaster [26]. Oocysts were not differentiated at the species level but designated as *Eimeria* spp.; they were counted microscopically, and the intensity of infection was expressed as oocysts per gram of feces (OPG).

### 2.7. Statistical Analysis

Treatment effects on the growth parameters, microbiota in fecal samples, and phagocytic activity (PA) were analyzed using two-way analysis of variance (ANOVA), followed by Bonferroni post-hoc test for pair-wise comparisons, where appropriate. Fixed effects for the model included period and treatment, and the interaction between them. Statistical analysis of microbiota from cecal and appendix samples, feed conversion and secretory IgA was performed with one-way analysis of variance (ANOVA), followed by Tukey's post hoc test or pair-wise comparisons, where appropriate. The statistical model included the time, treatment effects and their interaction. When the interaction was significant, Fisher's Least Significant Difference test (Fisher's LSD) was applied post hoc to determine significant differences among the means. Statistical analysis of the applied SE P3/Tr2a strain in fecal, cecal and appendix samples was performed using unpaired Student *t*-test. All statistical analyses were performed by the GraphPad Prism statistical software (GraphPad Prism version 9.3.1., GraphPad Software, San Diego, CA, USA). Differences between the mean values of the different dietary treatments were considered statistically significant at $p < 0.05$. Data are expressed as means and standard deviations of the mean (SD).

## 3. Results

### 3.1. Growth Performance of Rabbits

The animals were in good health throughout the experiment. Mortality was noted in groups S, E + S, and C (Table 2). Higher BW and ADWG were recorded in all experimental groups during additives' application compared to the control data (E: by 20.5%; S: by 17.1%; E + S: by 25.6%; Table 2). The highest BW and ADWG (E; $p < 0.0001$) and the lowest FCR (E: by 10.2%) were noted during Ent A/P application. Lower FCR (by 1.5%) was also noted in the E + S group, compared to C.

**Table 2.** Growth performance, phagocytic activity, and secretory IgA of rabbits.

| Tested Parameters | Day | E | S | E + S | C | *p*-Value | | |
|---|---|---|---|---|---|---|---|---|
| | | | | | | Time | Treatment | Time × Treatment |
| Body weight (g) | 0 | 1153.0 ± 178.2 [a] | 1140.2 ± 149.3 [ab] | 1060.9 ± 150.8 [ab] | 1012.9 ± 118.8 [b] | <0.0001 | <0.0001 | 0.2982 |
| | 14 | 1735.0 ± 260.0 [a] | 1734.5 ± 152.3 [ab] | 1691.5 ± 213.1 [ab] | 1487.8 ± 203.9 [b] | | | |
| | 21 | 2052.7 ± 266.1 [a] | 2014.8 ± 186.1 [ab] | 1999.0 ± 212.2 [ab] | 1759.7 ± 218.6 [b] | | | |
| Average daily weight gain (ADWG; g/day/rabbit) | 0–14 | 41.58 ± 5.85 [a] | 42.45 ± 8.67 [ab] | 45.04 ± 9.54 [ab] | 33.92 ± 8.53 [b] | 0.2940 | <0.0001 | 0.0997 |
| | 14–21 | 45.39 ± 8.13 [a] | 40.04 ± 8.82 [ab] | 43.93 ± 7.80 [ab] | 38.85 ± 10.61 [b] | | | |
| Mortality (rabbit/group) | 0–21 | 0 | 1 | 2 | 1 | | | |
| Feed conversion (g/g) | 0–21 | 2.37 ± 0.44 | 2.78 ± 0.92 | 2.60 ± 0.67 | 2.64 ± 0.20 | | 0.1493 | |
| Phagocytic activity (PA; %) | 0 | 63.75 ± 3.33 | 63.75 ± 3.33 | 63.75 ± 3.33 | 63.75 ± 3.33 | 0.0097 | <0.0001 | <0.0001 |
| | 14 | 69.63 ± 2.13 [Aa] | 61.63 ± 2.77 [Bb] | 71.00 ± 2.14 [Aa] | 59.63 ± 3.66 [Bb] | | | |
| | 21 | 70.25 ± 1.39 [Aa] | 81.13 ± 1.60 [Bb] | 53.88 ± 3.60 [Cc] | 58.25 ± 2.82 [Dd] | | | |
| Secretory IgA (µg/g) | 21 | 9.817 ± 0.765 [a] | 9.929 ± 0.635 [a] | 17.240 ± 3.694 [b] | 9.705 ± 0.761 [a] | | 0.0220 | |

E–Ent A/P application between 0–14 days; S–SE P3/Tr2a application between 14–21 days; E + S–Ent A/P preventive application for 2 weeks (between 0–14 days) before SE P3Tr2a strain addition for 1 week (between 14–21 days); C–control group (without additives); Data are expressed as means and standard deviations (SD). [a], [b], [c], [d] Means within lines with different superscript letters are significantly different ($p < 0.05$) using Bonferroni post hoc test; [A], [B], [C], [D] Means within lines with different superscript letters are significantly different ($p < 0.05$) using Fisher's LSD post hoc test. The bold letters mean significant changes.

### 3.2. Immunoglobulin A in Small Intestinal Wall and Phagocytic Activity in Blood

The time and treatment effect was noted on the PA in this study ($p < 0.0001$; Table 2). Ent A/P addition increased the PA values compared to C (day 14; E, E + S vs. C: $p < 0.001$); higher PA was noted one week after its withdrawal only in group E (day 21; E vs. E + S, C:

$p < 0.001$). The SE P3/Tr2a strain application to rabbits decreased PA in the E + S group after 2 weeks of Ent A/P addition (day 21; E + S vs. E, S and C: $p < 0.001$), but, on the contrary, the PA value was elevated in group S, without Ent A/P preventive application (S vs. E, E + S, C: $p < 0.001$). The interaction effect was noted at day 14 (E vs. S, C: $p < 0.0001$; E + S vs. E, C: $p < 0.0001$), and at day 2 (E vs. S, E + S, C: $p < 0.0001$; S vs. E + S, C: $p < 0.0001$; E + S vs. C: $p < 0.01$).

IgA levels were similar among the experimental groups, except the E + S group, showing the highest IgA value ($p = 0.0220$; Table 2).

### 3.3. Microbial Population

In feces, most bacteria were influenced by time, treatment, and their interaction (except amylolytic streptococci; Table 3). At day 14, lower counts of all tested bacterial groups, except MRS, were recorded compared to the initial data (day 0/1) and the highest count of coliforms, amylolytic streptococci, staphylococci, MRS, and total bacteria was noted in the S group on this day. At the end of SE P3/Tr2a strain application in the E + S group (day 21), a significant reduction of enterococci, coliforms, MRS (E + S vs. E, S, C: $p < 0.001$), amylolytic streptococci, and total bacterial count (E + S vs. E, S: $p < 0.001$) was detected. The time and treatment interaction was noted on coliforms already at day 14 (S vs. E: $p < 0.0001$; S vs. E + S: $p < 0.001$; S vs. C: $p < 0.01$). At the end of the experiment, enterococci (E + S vs. E, C: $p < 0.0001$; E + S vs. S: $p < 0.001$), staphylococci, and total bacteria (E vs. E + S: $p < 0.05$; S vs. E + S: $p < 0.001$; S vs. C: $p < 0.01$), MRS (E vs. S: $p < 0.01$; E + S vs. E, C: $p < 0.0001$; E + S vs. S: $p < 0.001$), and coliforms (E vs. E + S: $p < 0.05$; S vs. E + S: $p < 0.01$) were influenced by the time and treatment interaction.

**Table 3.** Bacterial counts (log 10 CFU/g ± SD) in feces of rabbits.

| Bacteria | Day | E | S | E + S | C | p-Value | | |
|---|---|---|---|---|---|---|---|---|
| | | | | | | Time | Treatment | Time × Treatment |
| Enterococcus spp. | 0 | 3.49 ± 0.30 | 3.49 ± 0.30 | 3.49 ± 0.30 | 3.49 ± 0.30 | <0.0001 | <0.0001 | <0.0001 |
| | 14 | 2.77 ± 0.86 | 2.51 ± 0.78 | 2.97 ± 0.38 | 2.43 ± 1.02 | | | |
| | 21 | 3.09 ± 0.41 [Aa] | 2.52 ± 0.49 [Ab] | 1.46 ± 0.69 [Bc] | 2.76 ± 0.53 [Aa] | | | |
| Coliforms | 0 | 3.59 ± 1.73 | 3.59 ± 1.73 | 3.59 ± 1.73 | 3.59 ± 1.73 | <0.0001 | <0.0001 | <0.0001 |
| | 14 | 1.17 ± 0.37 [Aa] | 3.61 ± 0.77 [Bb] | 1.60 ± 0.90 [Aa] | 1.67 ± 0.75 [Aa] | | | |
| | 21 | 2.26 ± 1.16 [Aa] | 2.68 ± 0.75 [Aa] | 1.00 ± 0.00 [Bb] | 2.14 ± 0.58 [ABa] | | | |
| Amylolytic streptococci | 0 | 3.94 ± 0.60 | 3.94 ± 0.60 | 3.94 ± 0.60 | 3.94 ± 0.60 | 0.4952 | 0.9087 | 0.9973 |
| | 14 | 3.59 ± 0.12 | 3.87 ± 0.53 | 3.22 ± 0.45 | 3.49 ± 0.30 | | | |
| | 21 | 3.76 ± 1.06 | 3.48 ± 0.62 | 3.16 ± 0.57 | 3.01 ± 0.74 | | | |
| Staphylococcus spp. | 0 | 3.87 ± 0.17 | 3.87 ± 0.17 | 3.87 ± 0.17 | 3.87 ± 0.17 | <0.0001 | <0.0256 | <0.0001 |
| | 14 | 3.65 ± 0.27 | 3.70 ± 0.26 | 3.55 ± 0.29 | 3.49 ± 0.30 | | | |
| | 21 | 3.30 ± 0.47 [Aa] | 3.02 ± 0.36 [Bb] | 3.67 ± 0.65 [Cc] | 3.60 ± 0.44 [ACc] | | | |
| Methicillin-resistant staphylococci | 0 | 2.38 ± 0.22 | 2.38 ± 0.22 | 2.38 ± 0.22 | 2.38 ± 0.22 | <0.0001 | <0.0001 | <0.0001 |
| | 14 | 3.65 ± 0.27 | 3.70 ± 0.26 | 3.55 ± 0.27 | 3.48 ± 0.38 | | | |
| | 21 | 4.01 ± 0.09 [Aa] | 3.55 ± 0.34 [Bb] | 3.06 ± 0.47 [Cc] | 3.79 ± 0.18 [ABd] | | | |
| Total bacteria | 0 | 4.96 ± 0.45 | 4.96 ± 0.45 | 4.96 ± 0.45 | 4.96 ± 0.45 | <0.0001 | <0.0001 | <0.0001 |
| | 14 | 3.09 ± 0.23 [a] | 3.59 ± 0.71 [b] | 3.45 ± 0.23 [bc] | 3.13 ± 0.44 [ac] | | | |
| | 21 | 3.92 ± 0.57 [Aa] | 4.37 ± 1.04 [Bb] | 3.38 ± 0.09 [Cc] | 3.65 ± 0.13 [ACac] | | | |
| SE P3/Tr2a strain | data | NT | 1.66 ± 1.20 | 1.20 ± 0.68 | NT | | 0.3615 | |

E–Ent A/P application between 0–14 days; S–SE P3/Tr2a application between 14–21 days; E + S–Ent A/P preventive application for 2 weeks (between 0–14 days) before SE P3Tr2a strain addition for 1 week (between 14–21 days); C–control group (without additives); Data are expressed as means and standard deviations (SD). [a], [b], [c], [d] Means within lines with different superscript letters are significantly different ($p < 0.05$) using Bonferroni post hoc test; [A], [B], [C] Means within lines with different superscript letters are significantly different ($p < 0.05$) using Fisher's LSD post hoc test. The bold letters mean significant changes.

The SE P3/Tr2a strain was able to colonize the digestive tract of rabbits after its one-week application, reaching counts in the range 1.20–1.66 log cycle in the feces (Table 3) and also in the range 0.90–1.00 log cycle in the cecum and appendix (Table 4).

Table 4. Bacterial counts (log 10 CFU/g ± SD) in cecum and appendix of rabbits.

| Bacteria | Source | E | S | E + S | C | p-Value |
|---|---|---|---|---|---|---|
| Enterococcus spp. | cecum | 1.63 ± 0.77 [a] | 0.90 ± 0.00 [b] | 0.90 ± 0.00 [b] | 1.56 ± 0.84 [a] | **<0.0001** |
|  | appendix | 0.90 ± 0.00 | 0.90 ± 0.00 | 0.90 ± 0.00 | 1.43 ± 0.41 | 0.0391 |
| Coliforms | cecum | 0.90 ± 0.00 [a] | 1.00 ± 0.17 [a] | 0.90 ± 0.00 [a] | 2.30 ± 0.67 [b] | **<0.0001** |
|  | appendix | 1.43 ± 0.91 | 1.39 ± 0.63 | 1.36 ± 0.49 | 1.05 ± 0.25 | 0.6810 |
| Amylolytic streptococci | cecum | 2.71 ± 0.44 | 3.35 ± 0.92 | 3.50 ± 0.67 | 2.93 ± 0.20 | 0.1091 |
|  | appendix | 2.96 ± 1.20 | 3.13 ± 0.94 | 3.18 ± 0.66 | 3.83 ± 0.70 | 0.2484 |
| Staphylococcus spp. | cecum | 3.02 ± 0.29 | 3.64 ± 0.36 | 3.29 ± 0.88 | 3.52 ± 0.45 | 0.1972 |
|  | appendix | 3.32 ± 0.20 | 3.65 ± 0.23 | 3.45 ± 0.16 | 3.17 ± 0.37 | 0.0952 |
| Methicillin-resistant staphylococci | cecum | 4.03 ± 0.50 [ab] | 4.17 ± 0.19 [ab] | 4.86 ± 1.77 [a] | 3.40 ± 0.27 [b] | **0.0489** |
|  | appendix | 3.40 ± 0.17 | 3.39 ± 0.23 | 3.52 ± 0.16 | 3.75 ± 0.29 | 0.2088 |
| Total bacteria | cecum | 3.22 ± 0.23 [a] | 3.73 ± 0.52 [ab] | 3.91 ± 0.35 [b] | 3.31 ± 0.20 [a] | **0.0188** |
|  | appendix | 3.73 ± 0.77 | 3.33 ± 0.25 | 3.50 ± 0.13 | 3.88 ± 1.22 | 0.1915 |
| SE P3/Tr2a strain | cecum | NT | 0.90 ± 0.00 | 1.00 ± 0.17 | NT | 0.9885 |
|  | appendix | NT | 1.00 ± 0.17 | 0.90 ± 0.00 | NT | 0.9885 |

E–Ent A/P application between 0–14 days; S–SE P3/Tr2a application between 14–21 days; E + S–Ent A/P preventive application for 2 weeks (between 0–14 days) before SE P3Tr2a strain addition for 1 week (between 14–21 days); C–control group (without additives); Data are expressed as means and standard deviations (SD). [a], [b] Means within lines with different superscript letters are significantly different ($p < 0.05$) using Tukey's post hoc test. The bold letters mean significant changes.

Most of the tested bacteria were enumerated in lower counts in the cecum and appendix (except cecal MRS), than in fecal samples. In the cecum, counts of enterococci and coliforms were reduced significantly ($p < 0.001$, Table 4) compared with C, while MRS and total bacteria were increased in the E + S group (E + S vs. E, C: $p < 0.001$).

Fecal samples in all groups (experimental and control) were *Eimeria* spp. oocytes absent.

## 4. Discussion

Good health status, higher BW, and ADWG of rabbits recorded in all experimental groups during additives' application indicated the beneficial effect of Ent A/P on the one hand, and on the other hand no negative impact of the SE P3/Tr2a strain on animals' growth was noted. However, reduced FCR in the E and E + S groups reconfirms the positive influence of Ent A/P on rabbits' growth performance, which can be explained by better feed intake and consumption; this finding is important from the economic point of view (less feed for faster growth). Faster growth and higher weight gain in rabbits were described in many studies during probiotics and their metabolites' application [27–30]. The beneficial effect of bacteriocins on the ADWG and FCR in rabbit experiments was repeatedly confirmed in this study, according to previous results [30–33]. The preventive effect of Ent A/P before SE P3Tr2a strain application to rabbits is reflected in the ADWG elevation and the FCR reduction compared to data from animals receiving only the SE P3/Tr2a strain, without enterocin treatment.

In addition to the positive impact of beneficial strains and/or their bacteriocins on animals' growth, their immunostimulatory effect is also important. These bioactive compounds can enhance immunity in several ways, including intestinal microbiota balance and the ability to modulate the host's innate and specific immune response. In general, stimulation of non-specific immunity is demonstrated by increased phagocytosis and modified cytokine production, while elevated immunoglobulins reflect the specific means of stimulation [34]. However, whilst several works have been published on the immune indices in healthy rabbits, existing knowledge on probiotics and bacteriocins' effect on phagocytic activity (PA) is still limited and needs to be expanded [35–37]. A significant increase of PA after 14 days of Ent A/P administration showed the non-specific immunity enhancement. Higher PA values noted one week after its cessation repeatedly confirmed the prolonged immuno-stimulative effect of Ent A/P, as it was previously described during several bacteriocins/enterocins treatment in rabbits [30,38]. The long term immuno-moderating effect of enterocins can be explained either by the maintenance of intestinal health, microbiota, and immunity via supporting the gut-associated lymphoid tissue (GALT), or by the adopting of animals on them. This finding also confirms the use of bacteriocins with a preventive effect in animals, compared to beneficial bacteriocin-producing strains, possessing immunoactivity already during their application and demonstrating more of the therapeutic effect of probiotics. The protective effect of Ent A/P was noted in the E + S group, as no increase in PA was noted after the SE P3/Tr2a strain application, while the strain itself without Ent A/P stimulated the rabbit immune system.

Several authors presented improved cell-mediated immunity [37] and an increased number of mast cells in the cecum, as well as higher IgM and IgG levels in serum [39] after probiotic administration to rabbits. It is well known that natural feed additives can stimulate immunity via enhancing rabbits' gut health. The predominant isotype of the mucosal immune system is the secretory IgA (sIgA), which can keep the mucosal immunity balance between commensals' microbiota and pathogens' defenses on the mucosal surface [40]. SIgA is synthesized by plasma cells in the lamina propria and translocated through intestinal epithelial cells, serving as the first line of defense to protect the intestinal epithelium from enteric toxins and pathogenic microorganisms by immune exclusion. Liu et al. [41] presented maintained intestinal barrier function and increased sIgA production after *Clostridium butyricum* probiotic administration to weaning rabbits, similarly to Plachá et al. [42] who detected a higher amount of IgA in the intestinal wall after thymol application to rabbits. In contrast to Chen et al. [43], who reported increased bile IgA in bacteriocin-treated broiler chicks, our results showed only slight (not significant) sIgA secretion after Ent A/P and SE P3/Tr2a strain application separately. On the other hand, SE P3/Tr2a application after preventive administration of Ent A/P significantly elevated the sIgA concentration. From this result, we assume that the higher amount of IgA detected in the intestinal wall is the result of the primary immuno-stimulation that is evoked by Ent A/P, and the secondary induced by methicillin-resistant SE P3/Tr2a strain as a possible agent. Given these initial results regarding the enterocin-protective effect, further studies on IgA secretion and mucosal immunity in rabbits are needed.

In addition to healthy intestinal immunity, a stable gut microbiome also contributes to the formation of animals' gut health. This microbial and immunological stability is often negatively influenced by several exogenous factors (stress, dietary and climate changes, etc.), but also can be improved mostly by natural feed additives, via strengthening the intestinal barriers, optimizing microbial balance, and supporting enzymatic activities and nutrient absorption in the gut. The in vivo antimicrobial effect of bacteriocins/enterocins in rabbits' gastrointestinal tract has been presented in several works [29,30,44–46], when mostly the counts of enterococci, clostridia, coliforms, and staphylococci were reduced. In rabbits, colibacillosis and clostridiosis are the main infections, particularly around the weaning period, when the animals are the most susceptible to these bacteria. Staphylococci as a part of the skin and mucosal barriers, and digestive tract as well, are also often detected as the main causative agents of skin lesions and abscesses and/or as associated pathogens in other multifactorial/multiorgan infections. Several works present the anti-staphylococcal activity of bacteriocins, including also MRS isolates [7,15,17]. While enterococci, coliforms and total bacteria were reduced at the end of Ent A/P application (14 days of the trial) compared to their initial data (day 0/1), balanced counts of tested bacteria within the experimental and control groups indicated no significant antibacterial activity of Ent A/P, including its anti-staphylococcal activity. These findings are contradictory to previously observed results during in vitro and in vivo enterocins' administration [15,30–33,45]. At day 21, at the end of SE P3/Tr2a strain application to rabbits, enterococci and coliforms significantly decreased in the E + S group, while staphylococci were noted in the highest counts; this fact may also indicate a possible competitive effect between the microbiota established in the gut and the applied SE P3/Tr2a strain. For this reason, we also expected a multiplication of the MRS bacteria, but, surprisingly, the lowest MRS counts were noted in the E + S group. On the other hand, this significant MRS reduction in the E + S group compared to negative (group C) and positive (group S) control at day 21 (after one week SE P3/Tr2a strain application) indicated the anti-MRS effect of Ent A/P, previously confirmed under enterocins in vitro testing against methicillin-resistant staphylococcal isolates [17]. The inhibitory effect on enterococci and coliforms was repeatedly confirmed in cecal samples of rabbits, similar to previous studies [30–33,45]. A significant increase of MRS and the total bacteria in the cecum, and their higher counts compared to fecal samples at day 21, can be explained as result of re-colonization with SE P3/Tr2a strain due to cecotrophy in the rabbits. To expand these results and already known facts concerning rabbits' health, immunity, and microbial balance by additives' supplementation is necessary through further investigations.

Coccidiosis is the most frequent parasitic disease in rabbit farms, affecting all ages, especially young, weaned rabbits, and causing high morbidity and mortality rates [46]. The oocysts are always present in the intestines of rabbits, and they cannot be eliminated even by the use of coccidiostat. Because the EU has banned antibiotics as feed additives and growth promoters, they are replaced with alternative anticoccidials, including prebiotics and probiotics, based on their bactericidal and/or bacteriostatic activities. Although *Eimeria* spp. oocytes were not detected in the feces of rabbits, the anticoccidial effect of Ent A/P can be expected, similarly to the anticoccidial effect of Ent 7420 noted in rabbits [30]; however, further studies are needed.

## 5. Conclusions

Good health and increased weight gain reflect the beneficial effects of Ent A/P on the growth performance of rabbits. These results also showed that the methicillin-resistant S. epidermidis SE P3/Tr2a strain did not have any pathogenic effect on rabbits' health status. The preventive effect of Ent A/P was recorded due to improved zootechnical parameters (elevated ADWG, reduced FCR), stimulated non-specific immunity (higher PA), and stabilized intestinal microbial environment (stable sIgA, reduced counts of coliforms, staphylococci, amylolytic streptococci, and total bacterial count as well) of rabbits. Reduced MRS and total bacteria after one week of SE P3/Tr2a strain application also point to the antibacterial effect of dipeptide Ent A/P and its anti-MRS potential. This study has an impact on basic research, confirming the in vivo anti-MRS activity of enterocin and also helping to spread knowledge regarding the interaction between intestinal microbiota and immunity.

**Author Contributions:** Conceptualization, M.P.S. and A.L.; methodology, Ľ.C., J.Š., V.F., I.P., Z.F. and M.C.; validation, M.P.S.; investigation, M.P.S., Ľ.C. and A.L.; resources, M.P.S.; data curation, Ľ.C. and M.P.S.; writing—original draft preparation, M.P.S.; writing—review and editing, M.P.S.; visualization, M.P.S.; supervision, M.P.S. and A.L.; project administration, M.P.S.; funding acquisition, M.P.S. All authors have read and agreed to the published version of the manuscript.

**Funding:** This research was funded by the Scientific Grant Agency of the Ministry for Education, Science, Research and Sport of the Slovak Republic and the Slovak Academy of Sciences VEGA, grant number 2/0005/21.

**Institutional Review Board Statement:** The study was conducted according to the guidelines of the Declaration of Helsinki and approved by the Ethics Committee of the State Veterinary and Food Administration of the Slovak Republic on 1 December 2016 (approval numbers SK CH 17016 and SK U 18016).

**Data Availability Statement:** Data available upon reasonable request to the corresponding author.

**Acknowledgments:** Part of the preliminary results regarding the growth performance was presented in the Slovak Journal of Animal Science, 2021, 54(2), pp. 57–65. We are grateful to G. Štrkolcová for *Eimeria* spp. oocysts analysis, to D. Melišová and P. Jerga for their skillful technical assistance and to J. Pecho for slaughtering. We are grateful for English language editing.

**Conflicts of Interest:** The authors declare no conflict of interest. The funders had no role in the design of the study; in the collection, analyses, or interpretation of data; in the writing of the manuscript, or in the decision to publish the results.

## References

1. Franz, C.H.M.A.P.; van Belkum, M.J.; Holzapfel, W.H.; Abriouel, H.; Gálvez, A. Diversity of enterococcal bacteriocins and their grouping in a new classification scheme. *FEMS Microbiol. Rev.* **2007**, *31*, 293–310. [CrossRef]
2. Soltani, S.; Hammami, R.; Cotter, P.D.; Rebuffat, S.; Ben Said, L.; Gaudreau, H.; Bédard, F.; Biron, E.; Drider, D.; Fliss, I. Bacteriocins as a new generation of antimicrobials: Toxicity aspects and regulations. *FEMS Microbiol. Rev.* **2021**, *45*, 039. [CrossRef] [PubMed]
3. Benítez-Chao, D.F.; León-Buitimea, A.; Lerma-Escalera, J.A.; Morones-Ramírez, J.R. *Bacteriocins:* An overview of antimicrobial, toxicity, and biosafety assessment by in vivo models. *Front. Microbiol.* **2021**, *12*, 1–18. [CrossRef] [PubMed]
4. Cesa-Luna, C.; Alatorre-Cruz, J.-M.; Carreño-López, R.; Quintero-Hernández, V.; Baez, A. Emerging applications of bacteriocins as antimicrobials, anticancer drugs, and modulators of the gastrointestinal microbiota. *Pol. J. Microbiol* **2021**, *70*, 143–159. [CrossRef] [PubMed]
5. Hernández-González, J.C.; Martínez-Tapia, A.; Lazcano-Hernández, G.; García-Pérez, B.E.; Castrejón-Jiménez, N.S. Bacteriocins from lactic acid bacteria. A powerful alternative as antimicrobials, probiotics, and immunomodulators in veterinary medicine. *Animals* **2021**, *11*, 979. [CrossRef] [PubMed]
6. Bemena, L.D.; Mohamed, L.A.; Fernandes, A.M.; Lee, B.H. Applications of bacteriocins in food, livestock health and medicine. *Int. J. Curr. Microbiol. App. Sci.* **2014**, *3*, 924–949.
7. Simons, A.; Alhanout, K.; Duval, R.E. Bacteriocins, antimicrobial peptides from bacterial origin: Overview of their biology and their impact against multidrug-resistant bacteria. *Microorganisms* **2020**, *8*, 639. [CrossRef]
8. World Health Organization. WHO Publishes List of Bacteria for Which New Antibiotics are Urgently Needed. WHO Jt. News Release. 2017. Available online: https://www.who.int/news/item/27-02-2017-who-publishes-list-of-bacteria-for-which-new-antibiotics-are-urgently-needed (accessed on 17 January 2020).
9. Werckenthin, C.; Cardoso, M.; Martel, J.-L.; Schwarz, S. Antimicrobial resistance in staphylococci from animals with particular reference to bovine *Staphylococcus aureus*, porcine *Staphylococcus hyicus* and canine *Staphylococcus intermedius*. *Vet. Res.* **2001**, *32*, 341–362. [CrossRef]
10. Bhargava, K.; Zhang, Y. Multidrug-resistant coagulase-negative Staphylococci in food animals. *J. Appl. Microbiol.* **2012**, *113*, 1027–1036. [CrossRef]
11. Igbinosa, E.O.; Beshiru, A.; Akporehe, L.U.; Ogofure, A.G. Detection of methicillin-resistant staphylococci isolated from food producing animals: A public health implication. *Vet. Sci.* **2016**, *3*, 14. [CrossRef]
12. Nascimento, J.S.; Ceotto, H.; Nascimento, S.B.; Giambiagi-deMarval, M.; Santos, K.R.N.; Bastos, M.C.F. Bacteriocins as alternative agents for control of multiresistant staphylococcal strains. *Lett. Appl. Microbiol.* **2006**, *42*, 215–221. [CrossRef]
13. Mathur, H.; Field, D.; Rea, M.C.; Cotter, P.D.; Hill, C.; Ross, R.P. Bacteriocin-antimicrobial synergy: A medical and food perspective. *Front. Microbiol.* **2017**, *8*, 1205. [CrossRef] [PubMed]
14. Wang, T.; Liu, M. The effect of bacteriocins derived from lactic acid bacteria on growth and biofilm formation of clinical pathogenic strains. *Int. J. Clin. Exp. Med.* **2016**, *9*, 7343–7348.
15. Lauková, A.; Strompfová, V.; Pogány Simonová, M.; Szabóová, R. Methicilin-resistant *Staphylococcus* xylosus isolated from horses and their sensitivity to enterocins and herbal substances. *Slovak J. Anim. Sci.* **2011**, *44*, 167–171.
16. Al Atya, A.K.; Belguesmia, Y.; Chataigne, G.; Ravallec, R.; Vachée, A.; Szunerits, S.; Boukherroub, R.; Drider, D. Anti-MRSA activities of enterocins DD28 and DD93 and evidence on their role in the inhibition of biofilm formation. *Front. Microbiol.* **2016**, *7*, 817. [CrossRef]
17. Pogány Simonová, M.; Maďar, M.; Lauková, A. Effect of enterocins against methicillin-resistant animal-derived staphylococci. *Vet. Res. Comm.* **2021**, *45*, 467–473. [CrossRef]
18. Lauková, A.; Strompfová, V.; Skřivanová, V.; Volek, Z.; Jindřichová, E.; Marounek, M. Bacteriocin producing strain of *Enterococcus faecium* EK13 with probiotic character and its application in the digestive tract of rabbits. *Biol. Bratisl.* **2006**, *61*, 779–782. [CrossRef]
19. AOAC. *Official Methods of Analysis of AOAC International*, 3rd ed.; Association of Official Analytical Chemists: Washington, DC, USA, 1995.
20. Van Soest, J.P.; Robertson, J.B.; Lewis, B.A. Methods for dietary fibre, neutral detergent fibre and non starch polysaccharides in relation to animal nutrition. *J. Dairy Sci.* **1991**, *74*, 3583–3594. [CrossRef]
21. Mareková, M.; Lauková, A.; Skaugen, M.; Nes, F.I. Isolation and characterization of a new bacteriocins produced by enviromental isolate *Enterococcus faecium* AL41. *J. Ind. Microbiol. Biotechnol.* **2007**, *34*, 533–537. [CrossRef]
22. De Vuyst, L.; Callewaert, R.; Pot, B. Characterization of the antagonistic activity of *Lactobacillus amylovorus* DCE471 and large-scale isolation of its bacteriocin amylovorin L471. *Syst. Appl. Microbiol.* **1996**, *9*, 9–20. [CrossRef]
23. Strompfová, V.; Marciňáková, M.; Simonová, M.; Gancarčíková, S.; Jonecová, Z.; Sciránková, L.; Koščová, J.; Buleca, V.; Čobanová, K.; Lauková, A. *Enterococcus faecium* EK13—An enterocin A-producing strain with probiotic character and its effect in piglets. *Anaerobe* **2006**, *12*, 242–248. [CrossRef]
24. Šteruská, M. Tests for the investigation of leukocyte function. In *Haematology and transfusiology*; Hrubisko, M., Šteruská, M., Eds.; Osveta: Martin, Czechoslovakia, 1981.

25. Nikawa, T.; Odahara, K.; Koizumi, H.; Kido, Y.; Teshima, S.; Rokutan, K.; Kishi, K. Vitamin A prevents decline in immunoglobulin A and Th2 cytokine levels in small intestinal mucosa of protein-malnourished mice. *J. Nutr.* **1999**, *129*, 934–941. [CrossRef] [PubMed]
26. MAFF—Ministry of Agriculture, Fisheries and Food. *Manual of Veterinary Parasitological Laboratory Techniques*, 3rd ed.; HMSO: London, UK, 1986; pp. 150–152.
27. Kalma, R.P.; Patel, V.K.; Joshi, A.; Umatiya, R.V.; Parmar, K.N.; Damor, S.V.; Chauhan, H.D.; Srivastava, A.K.; Sharma, H.A. Probiotic supplementation in rabbit: A review. *Int. J. Agric. Sci.* **2016**, *8*, 2811–2815.
28. Bhatt, R.S.; Agrawal, A.R.; Sahoo, A. Effect of probiotic supplementation on growth performance, nutrient utilization and carcass characteristics of growing Chinchilla rabbits. *J. Appl. Anim. Res.* **2017**, *45*, 304–309. [CrossRef]
29. Wlazło, L.; Kowalska, D.; Bielański, P.; Chmielowiec-Korzeniowska, A.; Ossowski, M.; Łukaszewicz, M.; Czech, A.; Nowakowicz-Debek, B. Effect of fermented rapeseed meal on the gastrointestinal microbiota and immune status of rabbit (*Oryctolagus cuniculus*). *Animals* **2021**, *11*, 716. [CrossRef] [PubMed]
30. Pogány Simonová, M.; Chrastinová, Ľ.; Lauková, A. Autochtonous strain *Enterococcus faecium* EF2019 (CCM7420), its bacteriocin and their beneficial effects in broiler rabbits: A review. *Animals* **2020**, *10*, 1188. [CrossRef]
31. Lauková, A.; Chrastinová, Ľ.; Pogány Simonová, M.; Strompfová, V.; Plachá, I.; Čobanová, K.; Formelová, Z.; Chrenková, M.; Ondruška, Ľ. *Enterococcus faecium* AL 41: Its enterocin M and their beneficial use in rabbits husbandry. *Probiotics Antimicrob. Proteins* **2012**, *4*, 243–249. [CrossRef]
32. Lauková, A.; Pogány Simonová, M.; Chrastinová, Ľ.; Gancarčíková, S.; Kandričáková, A.; Plachá, I.; Chrenková, M.; Formelová, Z.; Ondruška, Ľ.; Ščerbová, J.; et al. Assessment of Lantibiotic type bacteriocin—Gallidermin application in model experiment with broiler rabbits. *Int. J. Anim. Sci.* **2018**, *2*, 1028.
33. Szabóová, R.; Lauková, A.; Chrastinová, Ľ.; Pogány Simonová, M.; Strompfová, V.; Plachá, I.; Čobanová, K.; Vasilková, Z.; Chrenková, M. Enterocin 4231 produced by *Enterococcus faecium* CCM 4231 and its use in rabbits. *Acta Vet. Beograd* **2011**, *61*, 523–529. [CrossRef]
34. Maldonado, G.C.; Lemme-Dumit, J.M.; Thieblemont, N.; Carmuega, E.; Weill, R.; Perdigón, G. Stimulation of innate immune cells induced by probiotics: Participation of toll-like receptors. *J. Clin. Cell. Immunol.* **2015**, *6*, 1000283.
35. Fortune-Lamothe, L.; Boullier, S. A review on the interactions between gutmicroflora and digestive mucosal imunity. Possible ways to improve the health of rabbits. *Livest. Sci.* **2007**, *107*, 1–18. [CrossRef]
36. Deptuła, W.; Nied´zwiedzka-Rystwej, P.; ´Sliwa, J.; Kaczmarczyk, M.; Tokarz-Deptuła, B.; Hukowska-Szematowicz, B.; Pawlikowska, M. Values of selected immune indices in healthy rabbits. *Centr. Eur. J. Immunol.* **2008**, *33*, 190–192.
37. Fathi, M.; Abdelsalam, M.; Al-Homidan, I.; Ebeid, T.; El-Zarei, M.; Abou-Emera, O. Effect of probiotic supplementation and genotype on growth performance, carcass traits, hematological parameters and imunity of growing rabbits under hot environmental conditions. *Anim. Sci. J.* **2017**, *88*, 1644–1650. [CrossRef] [PubMed]
38. Pogány Simonová, M.; Lauková, A.; Plachá, I.; Čobanová, K.; Strompfová, V.; Szabóová, R.; Chrastinová, Ľ. Can enterocins affect phagocytosis and glutathione peroxidase in rabbits? *Cent. Eur. J. Biol.* **2013**, *8*, 730–734.
39. Wang, C.; Zhu, Y.; Li, F.; Huang, L. The effect of *Lactobacillus* isolates on growth performance, immune response, intestinal bacterial community composition of growing Rex Rabbits. *J. Anim. Physiol. Anim. Nutr.* **2017**, *101*, e1–e13. [CrossRef] [PubMed]
40. Mantis, N.J.; Rol, N.; Corthésy, B. Secretory IgA's complex roles in immunity and mucosal homeostasis in the gut. *Mucosal Immunol.* **2011**, *4*, 603–611. [CrossRef]
41. Liu, L.; Zeng, D.; Yang, M.; Wen, B.; Lai, J.; Zhou, Y.; Sun, H.; Xiong, L.; Wang, J.; Lin, Y.; et al. Probiotic *Clostridium butyricum* improves the growth performance, immune function, and gut microbiota of weaning Rex rabbits. *Probiotics Antimicrob. Proteins* **2019**, *11*, 1278–1292. [CrossRef]
42. Plachá, I.; Bačová, K.; Zitterl-Eglseer, K.; LAuková, A.; Chrastinová, Ľ.; Maďarová, M.; Žitňan, R.; Štrkolcová, G. Thymol in fattening rabbit diet, its bioavailability and effects on intestinal morphology, microbiota from caecal content and immunity. *J. Anim. Physiol. Anim. Nutr.* **2021**, *106*, 368–377. [CrossRef]
43. Chen, C.Y.; Yu, C.; Chen, S.W.; Chen, B.J.; Wang, H.T. Effect of yeast with bacteriocin from rumen bacteria on growth performance, caecal flora, caecal fermentation and immunity function of broiler chicks. *J. Agric. Sci.* **2013**, *151*, 287–297. [CrossRef]
44. Lauková, A.; Chrastinová, Ľ.; Plachá, I.; Kandričáková, A.; Szabóová, R.; Strompfová, V.; Chrenková, M.; Čobanová, K.; Žitňan, R. Beneficial effect of lantibiotic nisin in rabbit husbandry. *Probiotics Antimicrob. Proteins* **2014**, *6*, 41–46. [CrossRef]
45. Pogány Simonová, M.; Chrastinová, Ľ.; Kandričáková, A.; Gancarčíková, S.; Bino, E.; Plachá, I.; Ščerbová, J.; Strompfová, V.; Žitňan, R.; Lauková, A. Can have enterocin M in combination with sage beneficial effect on microbiota, blood biochemistry, phagocytic activity and jejunal morphometry in broiler rabbits? *Animals* **2020**, *10*, 115. [CrossRef] [PubMed]
46. Pakandl, M. Coccidia of rabbit: A review. *Folia Parasitol.* **2009**, *56*, 153–166. [CrossRef] [PubMed]

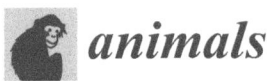

Article

# The Effect of the Season, the Maintenance System and the Addition of Polyunsaturated Fatty Acids on Selected Biological and Physicochemical Features of Rabbit Fur

Katarzyna Roman [1], Martyna Wilk [1,*], Piotr Książek [2], Katarzyna Czyż [3] and Adam Roman [4]

[1] Department of Animal Nutrition and Feed Science, Wrocław University of Environmental and Life Sciences, 25 C.K. Norwida St., 51-630 Wrocław, Poland; katarzyna.roman@upwr.edu.pl
[2] Independent Researcher, 51-649 Wrocław, Poland; pioksiazek@student.agh.edu.pl
[3] Division of Sheep and Fur Animals Breeding, Wrocław University of Environmental and Life Sciences, 25 C.K. Norwida St., 51-630 Wrocław, Poland; katarzyna.czyz@upwr.edu.pl
[4] Department of Environment Hygiene and Animal Welfare, Wrocław University of Environmental and Life Sciences, 25 C.K. Norwida St., 51-630 Wrocław, Poland; adam.roman@upwr.edu.pl
* Correspondence: martyna.wilk@upwr.edu.pl; Tel.: +48-71-320-5831

**Simple Summary:** Rabbit furs are a valuable material used in the fur industry. Many studies show beneficial effects of omega-3 acids supplementation on the skin and coat of animals. The aim of the study was to show the impact of environmental conditions and dietary supplementation with ethyl esters of linseed oil on the quality of the rabbit hair coat. The experiment was carried out in four stages: laboratory (summer and winter) and outdoor (summer and winter). The experimental rabbits were given an addition of ethyl linseed oil to their feed (during 2 months). To assess biological and physico-mechanical properties of the coat samples and to determine fatty acid profile and histological evaluation, the hair samples were collected three times: before the study, after two months of treatment, and after two months from the end of supplementation. The obtained results show that the environmental conditions have a major impact on the quality of the rabbit coat. The best results of hair heat protection were obtained from animals kept outdoors. Administration of linseed oil ethyl esters had a positive effect on the hair fatty acid profile.

**Abstract:** The aim of the study was to show the impact of environmental conditions and dietary supplementation with ethyl esters of linseed oil on the quality of the rabbit hair coat. The research was divided into 4 stages: laboratory (summer and winter) and outdoor (summer and winter). In each stage of the research, animals were divided into control and experimental groups. The animals were fed in accordance with the feeding standards of reproductive rabbits during the period of sexual dormancy. The rabbits from the experimental groups during the first two months were given an addition of ethyl linseed oil to the feed. In the experiment, linseed oil was cold-pressed directly in the laboratory. Three samples of hair were collected: before the study, after two months of treatment, and after two months from the end of supplementation. The hair coat biological properties, such as share of individual hair fractions (%), heat transfer index (HTI), hair diameter (μm), as well as physico-mechanical properties such as breaking force (N), breaking stress (kg/cm$^2$) and elongation (%) were performed. Moreover, the histological structure of hair and histological hair evaluation were performed. The fatty acid profile was determined in the hair as well. The obtained results of the content of individual fatty acids were grouped into saturated fatty acids and unsaturated fatty acids. In addition, omega-3 and omega-6 were distinguished from the group of unsaturated acids. The environmental conditions have a major impact on the quality of the rabbit coat. The best results of hair thickness and their heat protection were obtained from animals kept outdoors. The studies did not show an influence of the administered preparation on the quality of the rabbit coat. The hair became thinner, but more flexible and tear-resistant. Administration of linseed oil ethyl esters had significant, beneficial changes in the fatty acid profile in hair and hair sebum were observed. There was a significant increase in omega-3 acids, and a significant decrease in the ratio of omega-6 to omega-3 acids.

Citation: Roman, K.; Wilk, M.; Książek, P.; Czyż, K.; Roman, A. The Effect of the Season, the Maintenance System and the Addition of Polyunsaturated Fatty Acids on Selected Biological and Physicochemical Features of Rabbit Fur. *Animals* 2022, 12, 971. https://doi.org/10.3390/ani12080971

Academic Editors: Iveta Plachá, Monika Pogány Simonová and Andrea Lauková

Received: 14 March 2022
Accepted: 6 April 2022
Published: 8 April 2022

**Publisher's Note:** MDPI stays neutral with regard to jurisdictional claims in published maps and institutional affiliations.

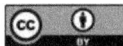

**Copyright:** © 2022 by the authors. Licensee MDPI, Basel, Switzerland. This article is an open access article distributed under the terms and conditions of the Creative Commons Attribution (CC BY) license (https://creativecommons.org/licenses/by/4.0/).

**Keywords:** rabbit; ethyl esters; linseed oil; fatty acids; hair coat

## 1. Introduction

Domestic rabbits (*Oryctolagus cuniculus f. domestica*), are the earliest domesticated fur animals in the world. The first attempts to domesticate European rabbits (*O. cuniculus*) consisted in keeping them in a semi-wild state, in specially separated and fenced areas (lat. *leporarium*) [1,2].

Two basic raw materials can be obtained from rabbits: meat—the so-called "white meat", and leather—for the production of furs, jackets, collars, and leather haberdashery [3]. The success in rearing and breeding rabbits is decided by many factors such as fashion, climate, and current demand for furs during a given season. Rabbit furs are an extremely valuable raw material used in the fur industry. Modern methods of fur and leather processing allow for the achievement of very good products with high market value. Compared to artificial furs, natural furs are fully biodegradable in mere years, which does not add to the pollution of the natural environment [4,5].

Nutrition is one of the base elements of rearing and breeding rabbits, which enables achievement of set production standards and effects. Rabbits are herbivorous creatures that require green feeds, root crops, and an appropriate amount of full-value concentrated feeds in order to achieve healthy growth. The base nutrition element, aside from protein and carbohydrates, is fat, that supplies fatty acids into the body. Their main division is made on the basis of the number of double bonds and distinguishes two basic groups: saturated fatty acids (SFA) and unsaturated fatty acids (UFA), which are divided into monounsaturated fatty acids (MUFA) and polyunsaturated fatty acids (PUFAs). The group of PUFAs can be divided into omega-3 (n-3) acids, which include extremely valuable α-linolenic acid (ALA) with its derivatives EPA (eicosapentaenoic acid) and DHA (docosahexaenoic acid), and omega-6 (n-6) acids, which include linoleic acid (LA) and its derivatives. The most important role for the human and animal body is played by omega-3 acids [6,7]. Neither acids from the ALA family nor acids from the LA family are synthesized in the human body and many animals, hence why they should be supplied from the outside with food [8,9]. Among the products of plant origin, the main source of n-3 acids are nuts, sesame seeds [10], linseed (about 50% ALA), and vegetable oils, e.g., soybean or rapeseed [11].

Linseed is an extremely rich source of valuable fatty acids. In seeds of traditional varieties, more than 80% of the sum of all fatty acids are PUFA, among which the vast majority is α-linolenic acid (about 60%). Thanks to this, the ratio of n-6/n-3 fatty acids in them is about 0.3. Linseed in meal form is given to livestock to enrich the feed with ALA. Many studies indicate that supplementation of animals with omega-3 acids has a beneficial effect on the skin and coat. Studies done on dogs have shown that the addition of linseed oil and linseed had a beneficial effect on hair growth rate and coat [12–14]. Small amounts of linseed are also added to feed for companion animals, e.g., songbirds and dogs, to improve the quality of plumage or coat [15]. Unfortunately, linseed also contains anti-nutrients such as linamarin and the enzyme linase that hydrolyzes it. However, the amount of linase and linmarine in linseeds can be reduced or completely removed through appropriate chemical processes, including the esterification process [15].

In this study, rabbits were used as model animals, in terms of research on the effect of omega-3 fatty acids on the state of the coat of fur animals. The aim of the study was to determine the effect of supplementation of the feed ration of rabbits with ethyl esters of linseed oil on selected features of the coat, including the profile of fatty acids. In addition, the conducted research was aimed at demonstrating the influence of changing environmental conditions, i.e., season and maintenance conditions, on selected physicochemical and biological parameters of the hair coat of termond white rabbits.

## 2. Materials and Methods

### 2.1. Animals

The experiment was conducted at the Wrocław University of Environmental and Life Sciences (Poland) and was divided into four stages (I, II, III, IV). Samples taken for the study consisted of hair coat samples obtained from rabbits of the termond breed kept in different systems during the summer (S) and winter (W), supplemented with the addition of ethyl esters of linseed oil. The tests were carried out in laboratory conditions (temperature approx. 18 °C, humidity approx. 65–70%), in single metal cages divided into boxes (I and II) and in production conditions, in external free-standing, two-story wooden cages (III and IV), equipped with a feeder and a droplet drinker. The cages met all animal welfare requirements and legal standards for keeping livestock [16].

For the experiments, males of the termond rabbit breed (about 3–4 months old) were used. Before the start of the study, all rabbits were examined by a veterinarian, dewormed, and then vaccinated against viral hemorrhagic rabbit disease and myxomatosis. After the adaptation period (2 weeks), the first samples were taken and ethyl ester supplementation began. Each stage of the experiment lasted 16 weeks: I-L-S (from June to September), II-L-W (from November to February), III-O-S (from June to September) and IV-O-W (from November to February). Feed administration continued for the first 8 weeks of each stage of the study. Hair coat samples were taken from the animals three times in each of the stages of the experiment: before the start of the study, 8 weeks after administration of the preparation, after another 8 weeks from the end of supplementation. After the end of the experiment, all rabbits were given for adoption to a private breeder.

### 2.2. Feeding

The animals were fed with a complete mixture, granulated (approx. 150 g of feed/day). The feed granules included: wheat bran, grass mixture, dried molasses beet pulp, sunflower post-extraction meal, rapeseed post-extraction meal, corn, alfalfa, beet molasses, post-extraction soybean meal (toasted), mineral-vitamin supplement. The percentage of nutrients in the feed was determined. Granules ingredients and chemical composition of granules shown Table 1.

**Table 1.** Ingredients (g/kg) and chemical composition of granules (g/kg of dry matter).

| Ingredients | | Composition | |
|---|---|---|---|
| Alfalfa | 205 | Crude protein | 166.3 |
| Grass mixture | 135 | Crude fiber | 148.2 |
| Wheat bran | 230 | Crude fat | 21.4 |
| Dried molasses beet pulp | 120 | Crude ash | 84.2 |
| Beet molasses | 100 | Calcium | 11.2 |
| Sunflower post-extraction meal | 60 | Sodium | 2.6 |
| Rapeseed post-extraction meal | 50 | Phosphorus | 9.7 |
| Corn | 40 | | |
| Post-extraction soybean meal (toasted) | 20 | | |
| Mineral-vitamin supplement * | 40 | | |

* calcium carbonate (20 g/kg), monocalcium phosphate (2 g/kg), sodium chloride (5 g/kg), sodium bicarbonate (25 g/kg), vit. A (8000 IU/kg), vit. D3 (1200 IU/kg), vit. E (25 IU/kg), vit. K (0.4 mg), vit. B1 (0.4 mg), vit. B2 (3.2 mg), vit. B6 (0.4 mg), vit. B12 (12 mg), biotin (80 mg), folic acid (0.45 mg), nicotinic acid (16 mg), pantothenic acid (6 mg).

All animals were provided with constant access to fresh water, hay and dried twigs from fruit trees (mainly apple and pear trees) [17]. The animals were fed in accordance with the feeding standards of reproductive rabbits during the period of sexual dormancy [18].

In the experiment, ethyl esters of polyunsaturated fatty acids obtained from linseed oil were used [19]. Linseed oil was cold-pressed, directly in the laboratory. A new batch of the test preparation was synthesized every 3 weeks. The preparation was stored in dark glass bottles in the refrigerator at 4 °C. Before starting supplementation with linseed oil ethyl esters, the addition of the preparation was tested on 10 rabbits not covered by experience for a period of 14 days. No disturbing symptoms were observed, e.g., loose stools, and the animals willingly ate feed with the preparation.

In the administered granulate, hay and ethyl esters of linseed oil, the fatty acid profile was determined (Table 2).

**Table 2.** Average fatty acid content of basic feed, hay and ethyl esters of PUFAs obtained from linseed oil.

| Acid | Hay | Feed | Linseed Oil Ethyl Esters | Acid | Hay | Feed | Linseed Oil Ethyl Esters |
|---|---|---|---|---|---|---|---|
| | Saturated fatty acids | | | | Unsaturated fatty acids | | |
| C6:0 | 0.57 | - | - | C14:1 | - | 0.07 | - |
| C8:0 | 0.66 | 0.02 | - | C16:1 | 2.33 | 0.32 | - |
| C10:0 | 0.64 | - | - | C17:1 | - | 0.05 | - |
| C12:0 | 1.26 | 0.03 | - | C18:1 | - | - | 16.73 |
| C14:0 | 2.4 | 0.12 | - | C18:2n-6c | 16.82 | 50.17 | 16.68 |
| C15:0 | - | 0.04 | - | C18:2n-6t | 17.66 | 21.32 | - |
| C16:0 | 28.83 | 15.39 | 4.44 | C18:3n-6 | 2.41 | - | - |
| C17:0 | - | 0.1 | - | C18:3n-3 | 5.3 | 5.9 | 58.71 |
| C18:0 | 4.98 | 4.24 | 3.43 | C20:4n-6 | - | 0.07 | - |
| C20:0 | - | 0.38 | - | C20:5n-3 | 1.75 | - | - |
| | | | | C22:6n-3 | - | 0.56 | - |

### 2.3. Arrangement of Experience

In all stages of the experiment, 16 rabbits were used, which were randomly divided into two groups: control (C) and experimental (E), 8 in each. Group C received granulated feed without additives, group E received an additional 5 mL of linseed oil ethyl esters per each animal for the first 8 weeks of the study, esters were administered in the morning, directly to slightly crushed granulated feed. All feed along with the dose of the preparation was quickly eaten, no leftovers were found. For the next 8 weeks, all animals were given feed without additives. The dose of the supplement was determined to achieve a tenfold reduction of the ratio of omega-6 to omega-3 EFAs in the rabbits' diet. The ratio of the above groups of acids after the addition of esters was about 1:1 (Table 3). This ratio of n-6:n-3 acids is considered the most favorable for the conversion of EPA and DHA from α-linolenic acid [20].

**Table 3.** Average content of omega-6 and omega-3 acids, and n-6/n-3 ratio in feed and esters.

| | n-6 Acids | n-3 Acids | n-6/n-3 |
|---|---|---|---|
| Basic feed | 72.03% | 6.46% | 11.15 |
| Linseed oil ethyl esters | 16.68% | 58.71% | 0.28 |
| Acid content in 5 mL of esters | 0.71 g | 2.50 g | 0.28 |
| Content in feed with added ethyl esters | 3.02 g | 2.71 g | 1.11 |

### 2.4. Physio-Mechanical Analysis of the Coat

The study evaluated the coat in terms of the share of individual hair fractions (%), heat transfer index (HTI), hair diameter (μm), physio-mechanical properties such as: breaking force (N), breaking stress (kg/cm$^2$) and elongation (%), histological structure of hair, fatty acid profile (%). The samples taken for determination of hair participation in individual fractions and heat protection were hair cast from an area of 25 cm$^2$ (5 cm × 5 cm) on the left side of the animal. Hair coat samples were taken once during each stage of the study, at the beginning of the experiment. The criterion for dividing hair into individual fractions was thickness, length and appearance. The above parameters were assessed using an illuminated laboratory lamp with a magnifier with a magnification of 20×. The amount of hair in individual fractions (%) was determined by separating the hair into down and ground cover hair using tweezers counting up to 1000 each sample. HTI was determined in two repetitions (about 2 g per each). The following formula was used to calculate the HTI:

$$HTI = HSD/HSDo = (M \times Cp \times R/A \times \alpha)/HSDo \qquad (1)$$

where: HSD—density of heat flux falling on the test sample (KW/m$^2$); HSDo—density of heat flux falling directly on the calorimeter (KW/m$^2$); M—the period of calorimetry (kg); Cp—specific heat of aluminum 900 (J/kg °C); R—the rate of increase in the temperature of the calorimeter in the linear part of the graph (°C/s); A—calorimeter area (m$^2$); $\alpha$—absorption coefficient of the blackened surface of the calorimeter.

In order to assess the effect of ethyl esters on the physico-mechanical parameters of the coat, the samples were taken three times: on the day of commencement of the study, after 8 weeks of administration of the preparation, two months after the end of supplementation. For measurements, hair combed out of the back of animals was used. Subsequently, measurements of thickness, elongation, breaking force, and breaking stress were made. The diameter measurements were made with an MP3 lamanester at a magnification of 500×, assessing 100 down hair and 100 ground cover hair from each sample.

The measurement of the breaking force needed to calculate the strength and elongation of the hair was performed on 30 randomly selected hairs, using the Matest electronic ripper and the computer program "Matest".

Measurements of the diameter and breaking force of the cover hair taken from rabbits during the research allowed us to calculate the value of the hair-breaking stress. This parameter is expressed as the ratio of the breaking force to the cross-sectional area of the hair.

$$N = P \times 10^4/\pi \times d^2 \times 9.81 \qquad (2)$$

where: N—breaking stress (kg/mm$^2$); P—breaking force (cN); d—diameter of the hair section (μm).

*2.5. Histological Analysis of Hair*

To assess the effect of the preparation administered during the research, photographs of hair taken immediately before the start of supplementation and after a two-month period of supplementation were taken. Hair obtained from rabbits from experimental groups was used for the analysis. Cover and down hair were evaluated. Histological evaluation was made using the LEO 435VO Zeiss scanning microscope (Carl Zeiss SMTAG). Based on the photos taken, the characteristics of the cuticle layer and their cross-section in down and cover hair were made. The slides for the photos were cleaned with ether and alcohol and rinsed in a sound scrubber for about 5 min, and after drying sprayed with gold. On the basis of the SEM (scanning electron microscope) images of down and cover hair at ×400, ×1000, ×2000 and ×3000 magnification, the arrangement of scales in relation to the longitudinal axis of the hair, the type of cuticle, the structure of the edges of the cuticles, the distance between the edges of the cuticles and the structure of the edges of the cuticles were determined.

*2.6. Fatty Acid Profile*

To investigate the effect of the administered preparation on the quality of rabbits' coats, the profile of fatty acids contained in sebum covering the hair was analyzed (7890A, Agilent Technologies, Santa Clara, CA, USA). The obtained results of the content of individual fatty acids were grouped into saturated acids (SFA) and unsaturated acids (UFA, including monounsaturated PUFA and polyunsaturated MUFA). In addition, two subgroups were distinguished from the group of unsaturated acids—omega-3 (n-3) and omega-6 (n-6).

Hair coat samples for the analysis of the fatty acid profile were taken three times: on the day of commencement of the study, after 2 months of administration of the preparation, and after two months from the end of supplementation. For measurements, hair combed out of the back of animals was used. Fat from rabbits' coats was extracted with ether by the Soxhlet method. Methyl esters of fatty acids were obtained according to the Christopherson–Glass methodology [21]. The fatty acid profile in the obtained samples was determined using a gas chromatograph (7890A, Agilent Technologies, Santa Clara, CA, USA) with an FID detector. The identification of the obtained fatty acids was carried out by comparison with the retention times of the standards of methyl esters of Supelco 37 fatty acids (Sigma Aldrich, Santa Clara, CA, USA).

*2.7. Statistical Analysis*

For each of the analyzed factors: additive—addition of linseed oil ethyl esters (C—control or E—experimental), condition—animal living conditions (L—laboratory or O—outdoor cage), and season—season of experiment (S—summer or W—winter), the tables present average values and standard deviation. The obtained data for main effects (additive, conditions, season) were analyzed by analysis of variance ANOVA using Statistica 13.3 (TIBCO Software Inc., Palo Alto, CA, USA). Significant differences between the groups were confirmed by Duncan's multiple range test. Highly significant differences at the level of $p < 0.01$ were marked uppercase—A, B and significant differences at the level of $p < 0.05$ were marked lowercase—a, b.

The obtained data for main effects were analyzed by analysis of variance ANOVA using Statistica 13.3 (TIBCO Software Inc., Palo Alto, CA, USA). Significant differences between the groups were confirmed by Duncan's multiple range test. Differences with $p < 0.05$ were considered as significant and $p < 0.01$ as highly significant.

## 3. Results

*3.1. Physio-Mechanical Analysis of the Coat*

Two fractions were distinguished from the tested control samples: cover hair and down hair. The ratio of both fractions was variable and depended on the season and where the animals were kept (Figure 1).

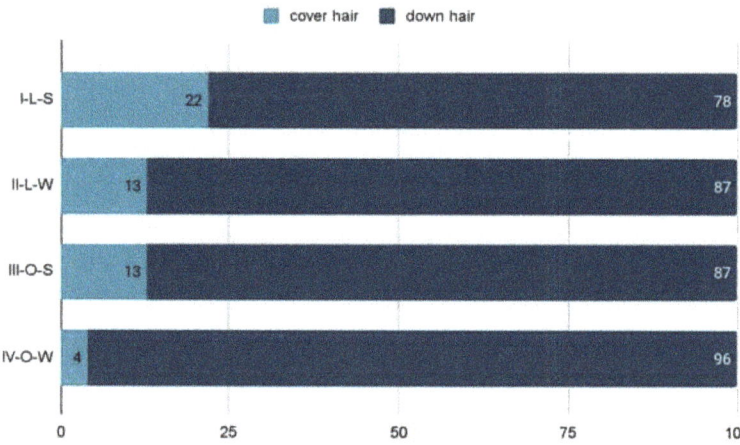

**Figure 1.** The proportion of cover and down hair (%) in the hair coat test—control group (L—laboratory conditions; O—external conditions; S—summer; W—winter).

Cover hair in the I-L-S group accounted for about 22% of the sample, and in the III-O-S group, about 13% of the sample. The down hair obtained at that time prevailed over the cover hair and accounted for 78% and 87% of the tested material, respectively. Studies during the II-L-W and IV-O-W periods showed that cover hair accounted for about 13% and 4% of the test material, respectively. As in the case of experiments carried out during the summer, down hair prevailed (87% and 96%, respectively).

Similarly, to the changes taking place in the proportion between cover and down hair, the HTI also changed (Figure 2). The coat of animals kept in laboratory conditions was characterized by much higher HTI values than in rabbits staying in external conditions. The lowest HTI value, and thus the best thermal insulation, was obtained during tests conducted in winter in outdoor conditions (HTI = 0.0435 W/mK).

The results of measurements of the diameter of down and cover hair are collected in Table 4.

**Table 4.** Impact of environmental factors (living conditions, seasons) and applied supplementation on chosen physicochemical characteristics of termond rabbit cover hair.

|  | Down Hair Diameter (μm) | Cover Hair Diameter (μm) | Down Hair Breaking Tension (N) | Cover Hair Breaking Tension (kg/mm$^2$) | Cover Hair Elongation (%) |
|---|---|---|---|---|---|
|  | mean ± sd | mean ± sd | mean ± sd | mean ± sd | mean ± sd |
| I-L-S C | 13.80 ± 0.51 | 73.54 ± 8.19 | 0.26 ± 0.02 | 1.69 ± 0.50 | 30.01 ± 1.90 |
| I-L-S E | 13.75 ± 0.58 | 62.48 ± 6.49 | 0.23 ± 0.03 | 2.12 ± 0.62 | 32.41 ± 3.27 |
| II-L-W C | 15.07 ± 0.66 | 68.52 ± 1.94 | 0.26 ± 0.02 | 1.92 ± 0.08 | 32.12 ± 0.35 |
| II-L-W E | 14.54 ± 0.52 | 63.11 ± 2.39 | 0.24 ± 0.01 | 2.13 ± 0.02 | 34.77 ± 1.72 |
| III-O-S C | 14.36 ± 0.51 | 66.25 ± 4.91 | 0.19 ± 0.01 | 1.39 ± 0.04 | 27.59 ± 3.37 |
| III-O-S E | 14.76 ± 0.10 | 67.56 ± 1.92 | 0.20 ± 0.01 | 1.55 ± 0.08 | 27.88 ± 1.10 |
| IV-O-W C | 15.28 ± 0.57 | 69.42 ± 0.68 | 0.23 ± 0.01 | 1.82 ± 0.10 | 31.02 ± 0.72 |
| IV-O-W E | 15.14 ± 0.31 | 68.93 ± 1.33 | 0.24 ± 0.00 | 1.64 ± 0.24 | 32.15 ± 0.87 |
| Additive | | | | | |
| C | 14.63 ± 0.78 | 69.43 [a] ± 4.99 | 0.23 ± 0.03 | 1.71 ± 0.30 | 30.19 ± 2.43 |
| E | 14.55 ± 0.64 | 65.52 [b] ± 4.26 | 0.23 ± 0.02 | 1.86 ± 0.40 | 31.80 ± 3.09 |
| Condition | | | | | |
| L | 14.29 [a] ± 0.75 | 66.91 ± 6.60 | 0.25 [A] ± 0.03 | 1.96 [A] ± 0.39 | 32.33 [A] ± 2.50 |
| O | 14.89 [b] ± 0.52 | 68.04 ± 2.67 | 0.22 [B] ± 0.02 | 1.60 [B] ± 0.20 | 29.66 [B] ± 2.60 |
| Season | | | | | |
| S | 14.17 [A] ± 0.59 | 67.46 ± 6.49 | 0.22 [A] ± 0.03 | 1.69 ± 0.44 | 29.47 [A] ± 2.99 |
| W | 15.01 [B] ± 0.54 | 67.50 ± 3.04 | 0.24 [B] ± 0.02 | 1.88 ± 0.22 | 32.52 [B] ± 1.69 |
| *p*-value | | | | | |
| Additive | 0.6883 | 0.0410 | 0.1127 | 0.2310 | 0.0618 |
| Condition | 0.0101 | 0.5304 | 0.0002 | 0.0088 | 0.0045 |
| Season | 0.0008 | 0.9818 | 0.0053 | 0.1351 | 0.0017 |
| Interaction | 0.9423 | 0.3058 | 0.7036 | 0.8086 | 0.8579 |

Experimental factor: Additive—addition of linseed oil ethyl esters (C—control or E—experimental), Condition—animal living conditions (L—laboratory or O—outdoor cage), Season—season of experiment (S—summer or W—winter), Interaction—interaction between all factors; [A, B]—highly significant differences at the level of $p < 0.01$; [a, b]—significant differences at the level of $p < 0.05$.

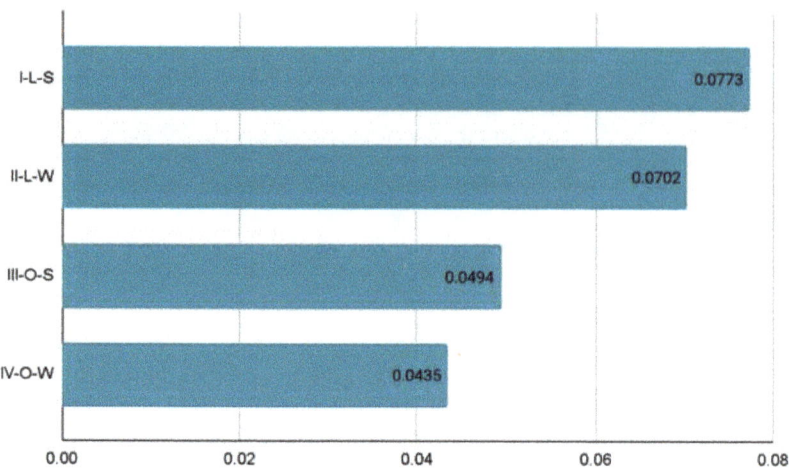

**Figure 2.** Heat transfer coefficient (W/mK) of rabbit coat—control group (L—laboratory conditions; O—external conditions; S—summer; W—winter).

The additive of linseed oil ethyl esters did not affect the physicochemical characteristics of termond rabbit cover hair except the cover hair diameter, which in the control group was statistically higher ($p = 0.0410$).

During experiment stages carried out in the laboratory condition, the lower down hair diameter ($p = 0.0101$) was observed compared to down hair diameter obtained from rabbits kept in outdoor condition. Moreover, during summer time, the rabbit hair was characterized by higher down hair breaking tension ($p = 0.0002$), cover hair breaking tension ($p = 0.0088$), and higher cover hair elongation compared to hair obtained from rabbits kept in outdoor condition. However, in both living conditions (laboratory and outdoor) the cover hair diameter was similar.

In animals kept during the summer time, the lower down hair diameter of rabbit cover hair was observed ($p = 0.0008$), and lower down hair breaking tension ($p = 0.0053$) and lower cover hair elongation ($p = 0.0017$) were compared to hair characteristics obtained from rabbit kept during winter time. However, the time of year did not influence cover hair diameter and cover hair breaking tension.

Statistical analysis did not show any interaction of experimental factors on the tested parameters.

*3.2. Histological Analysis of Hair*

Histological analysis of the hair showed that the cuticles of down hair were arranged longitudinally to the long axis of the hair. These were cuticles of the flaky, elongated type. The edges of all the cells of the cuticular layer were smooth. The cuticles of down hair were evenly distributed and arranged far from each other. Only one type of down hair was observed in all test animals (Table 5).

**Table 5.** SEM image of down hair of termond rabbits.

| SEM Image of the Cuticular Layer of Down Hair of Rabbits of Termond White Breed | |
|---|---|
| 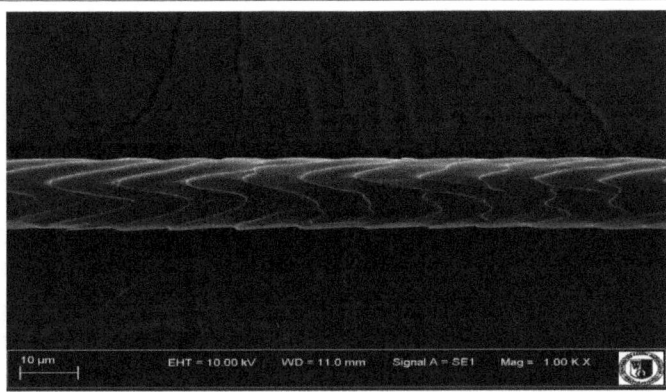 | |
| Period I-L-S | |
| Before supplementation | After supplementation |
| 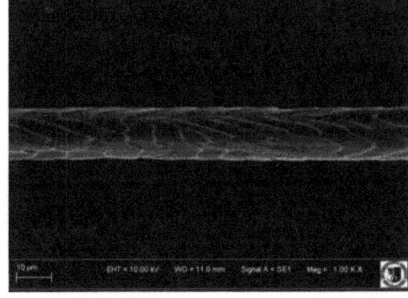 | 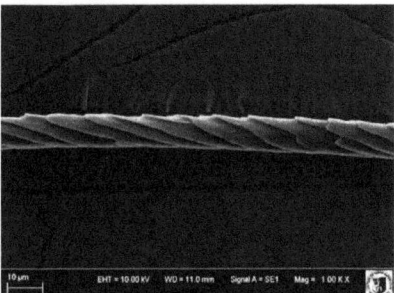 |
| Period II-L-W | |
| Before supplementation | After supplementation |
| 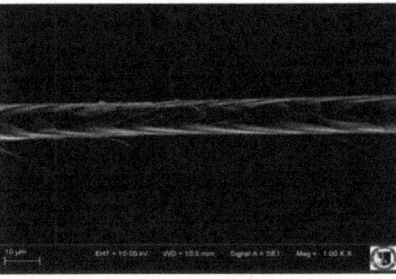 | 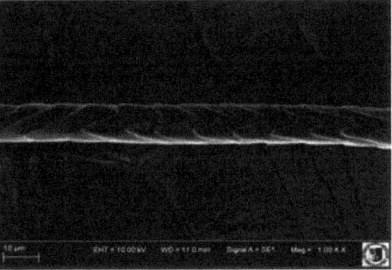 |

**Table 5.** *Cont.*

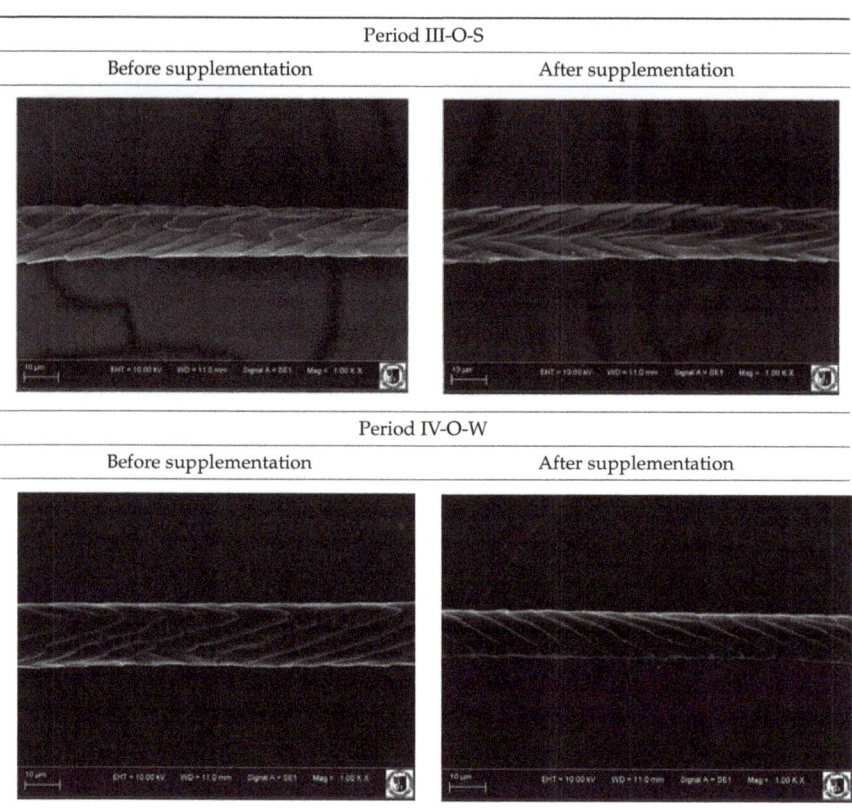

It was observed that the administered preparation with a high concentration of omega-3 acids improved the structure of down hair (a clearer drawing, optically greater smoothness of the epithelial-scaly layer).

The cuticular layer of the cover hair of rabbits of the termond white breed was characterized by two types of cell structure, depending on the place of their occurrence along the length of the hair (Table 6). In all cover hairs, the occurrence of the medulla was observed. It was a multicellular core whose cells formed an intermittent ladder pattern (Figure 3). It was shown that the cuticles located closer to the hair root were arranged transversely in relation to the longitudinal axis of the hair. Their shape was characteristic of the type of cuticles referred to as the broadly lobed type. The edges of these cuticles were slightly wavy and delicate irregularities on them could be seen. The distance between the edges of individual cuticles was small and even (Table 7). The cuticular layer located further from the root (closer to the top of the hair) were cells arranged longitudinally to the axis of the hair. The shape of these cells was characteristic of the elongated lobe type. The edges of the cuticles were smooth, devoid of any unevenness. The cuticles were arranged close to each other and partially overlapped (Table 8).

**Table 6.** SEM image of the cuticular lDayer of the cover hair of termond rabbits.

| The Part Located Closer to the Root. | The Part Located Further from the Root. |
|---|---|
| | |

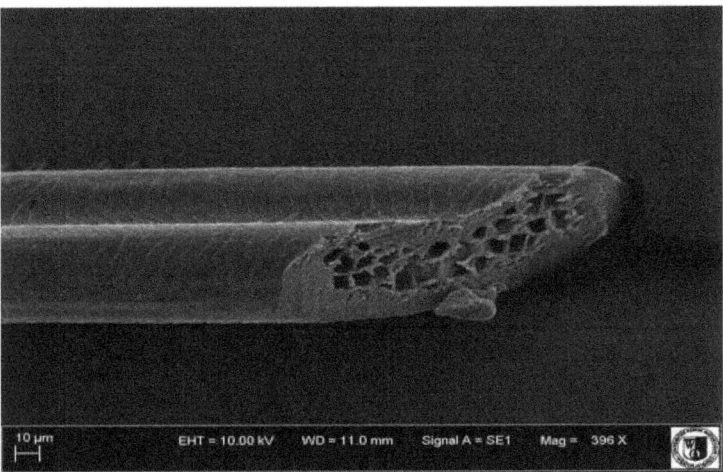

**Figure 3.** Cross-section of the cover hair of the termond rabbits—visible cells of the hair core.

**Table 7.** SEM image of cover hair (closer part) termond rabbits.

| Period I-L-S | |
|---|---|
| Before supplementation | After supplementation |
| | |

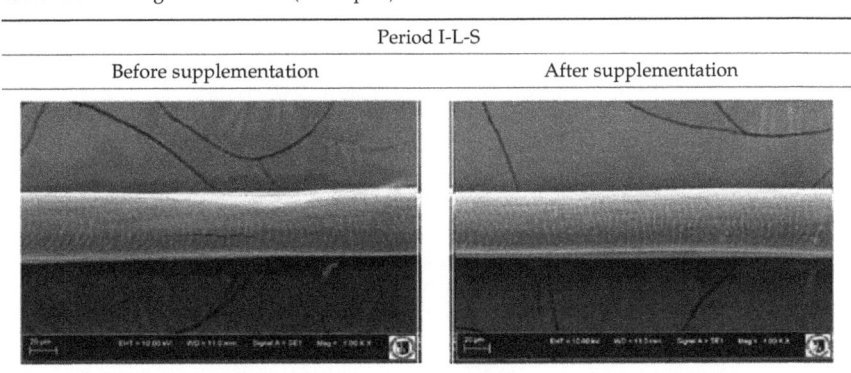

**Table 7.** Cont.

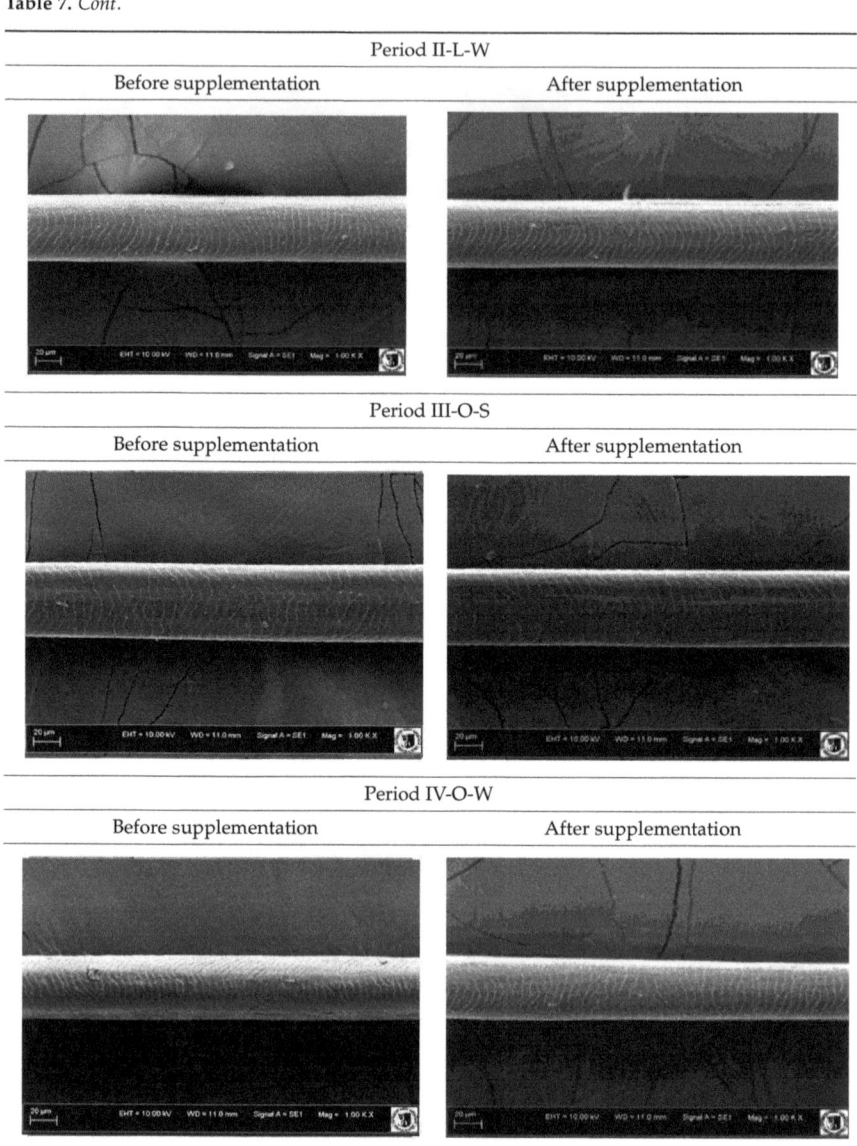

Analysis of SEM images showed no changes in the histological structure of the cover hair of termond rabbits. No modifications were observed in terms of the structure and arrangement of the cells of the cuticular layer both in the proximal part of the root and in the part closer to the top of the hair. A slightly clearer pattern of cuticles and a lower number of lesions on the surface of the hair after a period of supplementation were observed.

**Table 8.** SEM image of cover hair (further part) of termond rabbits before.

| Period I-L-S | |
|---|---|
| Before supplementation | After supplementation |

| Period II-L-W | |
|---|---|
| Before supplementation | After supplementation |

| Period III-O-S | |
|---|---|
| Before supplementation | After supplementation |

**Table 8.** Cont.

|  | Period IV-O-W | |
|---|---|---|
|  | Before supplementation | After supplementation |

### 3.3. Fatty Acid Profile

Statistical analysis showed a clear effect of the administered preparation on the fatty acid profile in the sebum of coat fur (Table 9).

**Table 9.** Fatty acid profile in rabbit coat sebum.

|  | SFA | UFA | MUFA | PUFA | N-3 | N-6 | N-6/N-3 |
|---|---|---|---|---|---|---|---|
|  | mean ± sd | mean ± sd | mean ± sd | mean ± sd | mean ± sd | mean ± sd | mean ± sd |
| I-L-S C | 46.95 ± 0.34 | 47.90 ± 0.40 | 28.30 ± 0.22 | 19.60 ± 0.26 | 1.02 ± 0.03 | 17.52 ± 0.21 | 17.21 ± 0.31 |
| I-L-S E | 44.79 ± 1.15 | 51.94 ± 3.69 | 29.51 ± 1.32 | 22.42 ± 2.38 | 2.94 ± 1.72 | 18.47 ± 0.64 | 9.47 ± 8.09 |
| II-L-W C | 48.58 ± 0.56 | 48.61 ± 0.16 | 27.41 ± 0.11 | 21.20 ± 0.13 | 1.53 ± 0.05 | 19.01 ± 0.11 | 12.49 ± 0.43 |
| II-L-W E | 45.51 ± 2.68 | 52.97 ± 3.75 | 28.98 ± 1.24 | 23.99 ± 2.52 | 3.38 ± 1.68 | 19.93 ± 0.88 | 7.43 ± 4.70 |
| III-O-S C | 46.00 ± 0.27 | 48.93 ± 0.51 | 28.92 ± 0.29 | 20.01 ± 0.24 | 1.69 ± 0.05 | 16.60 ± 0.12 | 9.91 ± 0.23 |
| III-O-S E | 41.55 ± 4.26 | 54.08 ± 4.68 | 30.68 ± 1.67 | 23.40 ± 3.02 | 4.06 ± 2.15 | 17.40 ± 0.60 | 5.73 ± 4.10 |
| IV-O-W C | 46.72 ± 0.24 | 48.90 ± 0.10 | 29.00 ± 0.07 | 19.91 ± 0.13 | 1.49 ± 0.01 | 17.40 ± 0.06 | 11.73 ± 0.10 |
| IV-O-W E | 41.86 ± 3.96 | 53.88 ± 4.73 | 30.39 ± 1.46 | 23.49 ± 3.27 | 4.11 ± 2.28 | 18.06 ± 0.72 | 6.20 ± 4.80 |
| | Additive | | | | | | |
| C | 47.06 [A] ± 1.04 | 48.59 [A] ± 0.52 | 28.41 [A] ± 0.68 | 20.18 [A] ± 0.66 | 1.43 [A] ± 0.26 | 17.63 [A] ± 0.92 | 12.84 [A] ± 2.83 |
| E | 43.43 [B] ± 3.32 | 53.22 [B] ± 3.72 | 29.89 [B] ± 1.41 | 23.32 [B] ± 2.48 | 3.62 [B] ± 1.76 | 18.46 [B] ± 1.15 | 7.21 [B] ± 5.04 |
| | Condition | | | | | | |
| L | 46.46 [a] ± 1.98 | 50.35 ± 3.18 | 28.55 [a] ± 1.13 | 21.80 ± 2.24 | 2.22 ± 1.44 | 18.73 [A] ± 1.03 | 11.65 ± 5.54 |
| O | 44.03 [b] ± 3.49 | 51.45 ± 3.88 | 29.75 [b] ± 1.26 | 21.70 ± 2.63 | 2.84 ± 1.87 | 17.36 [B] ± 0.67 | 8.39 ± 3.76 |
| | Season | | | | | | |
| S | 44.82 ± 2.85 | 50.71 ± 3.61 | 29.35 ± 1.13 | 21.36 ± 2.34 | 2.43 ± 1.69 | 17.50 [A] ± 0.79 | 10.58 ± 5.82 |
| W | 45.67 ± 3.29 | 51.09 ± 3.56 | 28.95 ± 1.37 | 22.15 ± 2.48 | 2.63 ± 1.70 | 18.60 [B] ± 1.11 | 9.46 ± 4.02 |
| | $p$-value | | | | | | |
| Additive | 0.0014 | 0.0017 | 0.0027 | 0.0014 | 0.0014 | 0.0012 | 0.0033 |
| Condition | 0.0207 | 0.3869 | 0.0111 | 0.9024 | 0.2944 | 0.0000 | 0.0629 |
| Season | 0.3842 | 0.7625 | 0.3427 | 0.3486 | 0.7347 | 0.0000 | 0.5030 |
| Interaction | 0.8958 | 0.9218 | 0.6673 | 0.9455 | 0.8945 | 0.9133 | 0.5447 |

Experimental factor: Additive—addition of linseed oil ethyl esters (control or experimental), Condition—animal living conditions (laboratory or outdoor cage), Season—season of experiment (summer or winter), Interaction—interaction between factors; [A, B]—highly significant differences at the level of $p < 0.01$; [a, b]—significant differences at the level of $p < 0.05$.

The additive of linseed oil ethyl esters influenced fatty acids profile in rabbit coat sebum ($p < 0.01$). The concentration of UFA (MUFA and PUFA) were statistically higher in the experimental group and the concentration of SFA was lower in the experimental group ($p = 0.0014$) compared to the control group.

During experiment stages carried out in the outdoor condition the lower concentration of SFA ($p = 0.0207$) and n-6 fatty acids ($p = 0.0000$) were observed compared to laboratory conditions. In contrast to concentration of MUFA, which was lower in samples collected from rabbits kept in laboratory condition ($p = 0.0111$).

Statistical analysis showed the influence of the season on the concentration of n-6 fatty acids, which was higher ($p = 0.0000$) in samples collected during the winter period of the experiment.

Statistical analysis did not show any interaction of experimental factors on the tested parameters.

In the n-3 acids group, ALA, EPA, and DHA and in the n-6 acids group, LA, GLA, and ALA were determined. In each stage of the study, the content of these acids significantly increased ($p < 0.01$) as a result of linseed oil ethyl esters supplementation (Table 10).

Table 10. Content of omega 3 and omega 6 fatty acids in the sebum of rabbit hair coat.

|   | Omega 3 Acids | | | Omega 6 Acids | | |
|---|---|---|---|---|---|---|
|   | ALA | EPA | DHA | LA | GLA | ALA |
|   | mean ± sd | mean ± sd | mean ± sd | mean ± sd | mean ± sd | mean ± sd |
| I-L-S C | 0.79 ± 0.02 | 0.13 ± 0.00 | 0.10 ± 0.01 | 16.90 ± 0.22 | 0.32 ± 0.01 | 0.29 ± 0.02 |
| I-L-S E | 1.31 ± 0.50 | 0.61 ± 0.44 | 1.01 ± 0.79 | 17.76 ± 0.79 | 0.44 ± 0.08 | 0.34 ± 0.02 |
| II-L-W C | 1.33 ± 0.05 | 0.10 ± 0.01 | 0.10 ± 0.01 | 18.10 ± 0.11 | 0.59 ± 0.02 | 0.32 ± 0.03 |
| II-L-W E | 1.99 ± 0.62 | 0.56 ± 0.41 | 0.84 ± 0.53 | 18.88 ± 0.74 | 0.65 ± 0.02 | 0.41 ± 0.13 |
| III-O-S C | 1.44 ± 0.05 | 0.13 ± 0.00 | 0.12 ± 0.01 | 15.92 ± 0.11 | 0.43 ± 0.02 | 0.24 ± 0.02 |
| III-O-S E | 2.41 ± 0.93 | 0.70 ± 0.51 | 0.95 ± 0.62 | 16.58 ± 0.52 | 0.45 ± 0.02 | 0.37 ± 0.06 |
| IV-O-W C | 1.26 ± 0.01 | 0.12 ± 0.01 | 0.11 ± 0.01 | 16.57 ± 0.06 | 0.52 ± 0.01 | 0.31 ± 0.01 |
| IV-O-W E | 2.57 ± 1.13 | 0.65 ± 0.47 | 0.89 ± 0.52 | 17.15 ± 0.65 | 0.55 ± 0.03 | 0.37 ± 0.06 |
| | Additive | | | | | |
| C | 1.21 [A] ± 0.26 | 0.12 [A] ± 0.02 | 0.11 [A] ± 0.01 | 16.87 [A] ± 0.83 | 0.47 [A] ± 0.11 | 0.29 [A] ± 0.04 |
| E | 2.07 [B] ± 0.87 | 0.63 [B] ± 0.39 | 0.92 [B] ± 0.60 | 17.59 [B] ± 1.06 | 0.52 [B] ± 0.09 | 0.37 [B] ± 0.07 |
| | Condition | | | | | |
| L | 1.36 [a] ± 0.56 | 0.35 ± 0.05 | 0.51 ± 0.06 | 17.91 [A] ± 0.88 | 0.50 ± 0.14 | 0.34 ± 0.07 |
| O | 1.92 [b] ± 0.87 | 0.40 ± 0.04 | 0.52 ± 0.06 | 16.55 [B] ± 0.58 | 0.49 ± 0.05 | 0.32 ± 0.07 |
| | Season | | | | | |
| S | 1.49 ± 0.76 | 0.39 ± 0.04 | 0.55 ± 0.06 | 16.79 [A] ± 0.81 | 0.41 [A] ± 0.07 | 0.31 ± 0.06 |
| W | 1.79 ± 0.78 | 0.36 ± 0.03 | 0.49 ± 0.05 | 17.67 [B] ± 1.02 | 0.58 [B] ± 0.05 | 0.35 ± 0.05 |
| | p-value | | | | | |
| Additive | 0.0024 | 0.0013 | 0.0012 | 0.0025 | 0.0011 | 0.0035 |
| Condition | 0.0324 | 0.7050 | 0.9715 | 0.0000 | 0.3874 | 0.4944 |
| Season | 0.2332 | 0.7798 | 0.7783 | 0.0005 | 0.0000 | 0.0788 |
| Interaction | 0.8457 | 0.9653 | 0.8770 | 0.9935 | 0.1919 | 0.2421 |

Experimental factor: Additive—addition of linseed oil ethyl esters (control or experimental), Condition—animal living conditions (laboratory or outdoor cage), Season—season of experiment (summer or winter), Interaction—interaction between factors; [A, B]—highly significant differences at the level of $p < 0.01$; [a, b]—significant differences at the level of $p < 0.05$.

During experiment stages carried out in the outdoor condition, higher concentration of ALA ($p = 0.0324$) and lower concentration of LA ($p = 0.0000$) were obtained compared to laboratory conditions.

Statistical analysis showed the influence of the season on the concentration of n-6 fatty acids (LA and GLA), which was higher ($p < 0.01$) in samples collected during the winter period of the experiment.

In the experimental group (with linseed oil ethyl esters) the increase of ALA content in the sebum of rabbit hair coat was 71% compared to the control group, while EPA and DHA showed an increase of about 425% and 736%, respectively. Supplementation of ethyl esters of linseed oil also had a significant impact on the level of omega-6 acids such as LA (+4%), GLA (+11%), ALA (+28%) in the sebum of rabbit hair coat.

Statistical analysis did not show any interaction of experimental factors on the tested parameters.

## 4. Discussion

The share of various types of hair in the coat, and thus also the density of the coat, is one of the most important parameters determining the quality of the coat [22]. Figure 1 shows clear differences in the percentage of each hair fraction taking into account the season and conditions of maintenance. In animals kept in external conditions (III-O, IV-O), there was much more down hair, which was caused by the instability of weather conditions (ex. different temperatures between day and night), and consequently the need for better thermal insulation of the body. This difference is obvious due to the need for much greater insulation of the coat during low temperatures. In rabbits in laboratory conditions (I-L, II-L), a much larger amount of cover hair was obtained, due to stable, higher temperatures in the room. However, despite unchanged environmental conditions prevailing in the animal house, both in summer and in winter, rabbits underwent a molting process, changing the coat from "summer" to "winter". Most likely, this was due to the shortening light day, which was the only determinant of the change of season for animals kept indoors.

Hair of animals kept under changing conditions of the external environment (III-O, IV-O) was more susceptible to rupture and damage than that obtained from animals in laboratory conditions (I-L, II-L). In addition, higher breaking stress values observed in the experimental groups compared to the control groups (stages: I-L-S, II-L-W and III-O-S) may suggest a positive effect of supplementation of ethyl esters of linseed oil on the tested cover hair feature, however this was not statistically confirmed.

The heat transfer index is a measure of the heat passing through a sample exposed to thermal radiation. The lower the HTI value, the better the insulator the test material is. In the case of animals, better insulation of the coat means better keeping heat on the animal's skin, which in turn causes the animal to maintain the desired body temperature. In addition, increased heat protection also means that excess heat from the outside does not pass into the animal's skin, which in turn protects the body from overheating during hot weather. The coat of animals kept in laboratory conditions (I-L, II-L) was characterized by a much higher heat transfer coefficient than rabbits staying in external conditions (III-O, IV-O), which means weaker insulation of the coat, and consequently weaker thermal protection of the body. This was due to stable environmental conditions in the room, and above all higher and constant temperature and constant air humidity. In external conditions, the HTI value was much lower, i.e., the hair cover showed greater insulating properties and the animals did not freeze, despite different temperature and air humidity values. The lowest HTI value, and thus the best thermal insulation, was obtained during tests conducted in winter in outdoor conditions (HTI = 0.0435 W/mK).

Heat protection is one of the parameters determining the comfort of using fiber products. This feature is influenced by, among others, the type of hair fibers, their structure as well as the properties of the yarn, and the structure of the fabric made from the hair fibers in question [23]. The thermal insulation of materials is important due to the fact that it determines their purpose [24]. The available literature lacks research on the heat-insulating properties of rabbit wool. According to Żyliński [25], the heat protection of wool and woolen materials such as non-woven fabrics and knitted fabrics is in the range of 0.0440–0.0528 W/mK and is lower compared to vegetable fibers. This fact may indicate better insulating properties of materials made of fibers of animal origin. In a study conducted by Bucişcanu [26], thermal conductivity values for sheep's wool were obtained at the level of 0.037 W/mK. In turn, Hansen et al. [24] and Ye et al. [27] report that the thermal conductivity for wool can be 0.047–0.049 W/mK, depending on the moisture level.

The heat protection of the fabric is due to the insulation of the air between the fibers and the yarn. Fabrics made of straight fiber yarn quickly release heat by conduction when placed next to the skin. On the other hand, hairy fiber fabrics, due to the air insulation between the fabric fibers and the skin, retain body temperature [28]. Studies aimed at assessing and analyzing the thermal comfort of fabrics investigated the relationship between the type of fibers and the composition of fabrics and thermal comfort [28–30]. In these studies, it was shown that both the composition of the fibers and the structure of the fabric made of them have a significant impact on the thermal properties and moisture transfer of tested textile materials. It has also been shown that the properties of fibers have an impact on the subjective feelings of users of clothing made from fibers. According to Sirvydas et al. [29], the thermal comfort of the fabric is determined by the thickness, parameters regarding water absorption, and thermal conductivity. In turn, the thermal resistance of clothing as a set of textile materials depends on the thickness and porosity of individual layers, but since the changes in porosity of standard textile materials used in the production of clothing are not large, the total thermal resistance of clothing really depends on the thickness of the material [30].

Hair thickness is one of the most important features that characterize the hair fiber in terms of suitability for further processing [31,32]. The most useful for the production of high-quality yarn are thin, coreless fibers [33–35]. The experiment has not proven the effect of administering ethyl esters of linseed oil on the thickness of down hair. Both down and cover hair of animals kept in outdoor conditions were much thicker than down hair of animals in laboratory conditions. Research on the thickness of rabbits' coat was carried out by among others Khalil et al. [36]. The authors studied the cover of New Zealand and Californian rabbits and in the case of both breeds noted thickness of down hair in the range of 12–18 µm and cover hair in the range of 62–89 µm, depending on the age of the animals—the older the larger the hair diameter. This may explain the statistically higher values of down hair diameter obtained from animals kept in winter (i.e., older rabbits). Taha et al. [37], based on the diameter of the hair follicles, analyzed the diameter of the hair fibers of the Gabali rabbits, New Zealand white and Rex, and obtained results of approx. 35, 48, and 36 µm for primary follicles and 8, 14, and 13 µm for secondary follicles, respectively. In turn, wool derived from Angora rabbits is one of the most delicate animal fibers used in the textile industry. The thickness of down fibers of Angora rabbit wool ranges from approx. 7 to 16 µm, depending on many factors, such as age, gender, and environment [32,38,39], while the thickness of core hair can reach approx. 65 µm [40]. The results obtained in these studies for down hair are at the top of this range, while the results obtained for cover hair are slightly higher. However, it should be remembered that Angora rabbits, unlike the termond rabbits used in the experiment, are a breed typically used in wool production. In addition, according to Taha et al. [37], the most important feature to be taken into account when assessing the cover is its smoothness, which largely depends on the diameter of the fiber. Thick fibers can cause irritation when in contact with the skin. Therefore, an increase in the diameter of the fibre in the case of rabbit cover intended for use in the textile industry is considered an undesirable feature. Beroual et al. [41] conducted a study in which they analyzed the effect of adding flax grain into rabbit feed and rubbing linseed oil into the skin on hair growth and thickness. The authors observed that rubbing linseed oil had an effect on hair thickness, which in the experimental group increased after 4 weeks of the experiment by about 44% compared to the control group. Feeding flax seeds with feed led to different results, in the initial stage it caused a decrease in hair thickness, while an increase in this parameter was observed after 16 weeks of the experiment. However, it is worth noting that giving flax with food as well as rubbing linseed oil into the skin had a beneficial effect on hair growth and mass. The authors suggest that α-linolenic acid (ALA) contained in flaxseed oil and linseed oil may inhibit the activity of 5-α-reductase, the enzyme responsible for converting testosterone to dihydrotestosterone. This hormone causes hair follicle shrinkage and changes in the hair cycle, so inhibition of its formation may explain the beneficial effect of flax on the coat [41].

The breaking force is the force to be applied in order to obtain maximum possible elongation value without the disruption of continuity of fibres of plant or animal origin, including hair. Its study is aimed at determining the tensile strength of the material. The higher the force needed to tear the hair, the more flexible and resistant to damage it is. Breaking stress, like breaking force, is one of the determinants of the quality of an animal hair coat, by determining the elasticity and resistance of hair to mechanical damage. Mengüç et al. [39] report that the hair elongation of the Angora rabbit is in the range of approx. 40–57%, which is definitely higher than the results obtained in their own research. In turn, the elongation values obtained in studies conducted by Wyrostek et al. [42] on the coat of cats was in the range from 10% to 32% depending on the type of hair and the color of the coat (higher values were obtained for dark cover), while in horse hair this parameter ranged from approx. 44% to 55% depending on the breed of horse and type of hair [43]. In turn, the breaking stress values obtained in these studies were about 2–3 times lower compared to the coat of cats or fur animals, in which this parameter was at the level of approx. 4–7 kg/mm$^2$, and definitely lower than the values obtained for the cover of dogs or sheep (about 15 kg/mm$^2$) [44,45].

The physio-mechanical properties of hair fibers are extremely important and determine suitability in the textile industry and purpose, testify to the condition of the hair, and thus indirectly also to the condition and health of animals [43,46,47]. One of the most important factors affecting the strength of fibers is air humidity: at higher values the fiber is more stretchable, because water acts as a plasticizing agent, while dry fibers, thanks to hydrogen bonds, are resistant to elongation. A similar effect was observed for temperature, as it increases, the hair fiber is weaker and more prone to stretching. An additional factor affecting the reduction of fiber strength are various types of acidic and alkaline substances [48]. The physical characteristics of rabbit hair were decisively influenced by the environmental conditions in which the animals lived and the time of year.

The hair of all animal species is characterized by a similar cellular structure, consisting of the medulla (which is not always found in down hair), a cortical layer, and a cuticular layer. However, the detailed structure of the individual layers is a genetically determined feature, characteristic of each species. The most diverse is the cuticular layer. Thanks to such characteristics as the shape and arrangement of cuticles, the appearance of the edges of cuticles and their distance from each other, it is possible to identify the species of animal, even after many years, which is commonly used, for example, in forensic science and archaeology. The arrangement and shape of the cover cells is also a characteristic feature of a given animal species [49,50]. The histological structure in terms of the arrangement of cuticles of the outer layer of rabbit hair, as well as the medulla obtained in own research, is consistent with the breed standard and data presented in the literature [51,52].

Ethyl esters of linseed oil are a rich source of many valuable fatty acids, especially those from the omega-3 group [19]. In order to investigate the effect of the administered preparation on the quality of rabbits' coat, the profile of fatty acids contained in sebum covering the hair was analyzed. The fat found on the hair is produced by the sebaceous glands and covers each hair with a thin, waterproof layer. Its main role is to protect hair from damage and water loss, as well as their nutrition [53]. Sinclair et al. [54] suggest that α-linolenic acid can enter the surface of hair fibers through the sebaceous glands and has a protective function against damage to the hair by water, light, or other harmful factors. Studies have also shown that ALA can be a factor in improving the growth of the coat. It was also observed that a diet low in ALA and rich in LA acid caused skin changes and hair loss. Changes in the ratio of SFA to UFA, especially an increase in the share of omega-3 acids and a decrease in the ratio of n-6: n-3 acids are therefore important in the context of improving protective properties by better moisturizing the hair surface [55,56]. MUFA, i.e., linoleic acid and α-linolenic acids, belong to the so-called essential fatty acids, which the body is not able to synthesize de novo and therefore must be supplied with the diet. These acids are precursors of subsequent long-chain fatty acids, which are biosynthesized with the participation of enzymes in processes involving elongation and desaturation. Both precursors compete for the same enzyme, D6-desaturase, which has a greater affinity for linolenic acid, which is why an adequate supply of α-linolenic acid is so important [57,58]. However, a controversial issue is the effectiveness of epa synthesis, and especially DHA from α-linolenic acid, which according to literature data is low and amounts to only about 6% and 3.4%, respectively [57,59–62]. This phenomenon is associated with the final stage of the DHA biosynthesis pathway, β-oxidation of C24:6n-3, which involves translocation between the endoplasmic reticulum and the peroxisomes of DHA and its precursor (C24:6n-3) [57,63].

Research in the field of nutritional modification of the fatty acid profile in rabbits and other livestock species was carried out mainly in terms of the quality of their meat [64–66], which is in line with current trends in functional food. However, it is also worth bearing in mind the aspect of animal health related to the activity of fatty acids from the omega-3 family, especially ALA as a precursor of EPA and DHA. In this study, rabbits were used as model animals, in the aspect of studies on the effect of omega-3 fatty acids on the state of the hair cover of fur animals [67]. As a result of supplementation, significant, beneficial changes in the fatty acid profile in hair sebum were observed. A significant increase in omega-3 acids, and a significant decrease in the ratio of omega-6 to omega-3 acids was observed.

## 5. Conclusions

Rabbits bred for fur should be kept in outdoor conditions, as is the case with other fur animals such as common and arctic foxes or American mink. Histological analysis of the hair of termond rabbits showed a variation in the structure of the cuticle depending on the type of hair. In the case of cover hair, the structure of the cuticular layer was also differentiated depending on the place of hair examination. The applied preparation of ethyl esters of linseed oil had a positive effect on the histological image of hair visible in a clearer drawing of cuticles and significantly higher strength. As a result of supplementation, significant, beneficial changes in the fatty acid profile in hair sebum were observed. There was a significant increase in omega-3 acids, and a significant decrease in the ratio of omega-6 to omega-3 acids.

**Author Contributions:** Conceptualization, K.R. and K.C.; methodology, K.R. and M.W.; software, K.R.; validation, M.W. and A.R.; formal analysis, K.R., M.W. and P.K.; investigation, K.R.; data curation, K.R. and M.W.; writing—original draft, K.R., M.W. and P.K.; writing—review, A.R. All authors have read and agreed to the published version of the manuscript.

**Funding:** The research is financed by Wrocław University of Environmental and Life Sciences.

**Institutional Review Board Statement:** The animal study protocol was approved by the Ethics Committee of Wrocław University of Environmental and Life Sciences (protocol code: 44/2015 and date of approval: 15 April 2015) for studies involving animals.

**Informed Consent Statement:** Not applicable.

**Data Availability Statement:** Not applicable.

**Conflicts of Interest:** The authors declare no conflict of interest.

## References

1. Rommers, J.; Meijerhof, R.; Noordhuizen, J.; Kemp, B. Effect of different feeding levels during rearing and age at first insemination on body development, body composition, and puberty characteristics of rabbit does. *World Rabbit Sci.* **2010**, *9*, 101–108. [CrossRef]
2. Carneiro, M.; Afonso, S.; Geraldes, A.; Garreau, H.; Bolet, G.; Boucher, S.; Tircazes, A.; Queney, G.; Nachman, M.W.; Ferrand, N. The Genetic Structure of Domestic Rabbits. *Mol. Biol.* **2011**, *28*, 1801–1816. [CrossRef] [PubMed]
3. Kanuri, W.D.; Onyuka, A.; Tanui, R. An Investigation on the Properties of Rabbit Leather from Different Tannages. *Int. J. Sci. Res. Publ.* **2019**, *9*, 12–17.
4. Saravana Bhavan, S.; Thanikaivelan, P.; Raghava Rao, J.; Unni Nair, B.; Ramasami, T. Natural Leathers from Natural Materials: Progressing toward a New Arena in Leather Processing. *Environ. Sci. Technol.* **2004**, *38*, 871–879. [CrossRef] [PubMed]
5. Sudha, T.B.; Thanikaivelan, P.; Aaron, K.P.; Krishnaraj, K.; Chandrasekaran, B. Comfort, chemical, mechanical, and structural properties of natural and synthetic leathers used for apparel. *J. Appl. Polym. Sci.* **2009**, *114*, 1761–1767. [CrossRef]
6. Spiller, G.A. *Handbook of Lipids in Human Nutrition*; CRC Press: New York, NY, USA, 1996.
7. Marciniak-Łukasiak, K. Rola i znaczenie kwasów tłuszczowych omega-3. *Żywność Nauka Technologia Jakość* **2011**, *6*, 24–35.
8. Kolanowski, W. Bioavailability of omega-3 PUFA from foods enriched with fish oil—A mini review. *Pol. J. Food Nutr. Sci.* **2005**, *14/55*, 335–340.
9. Flachs, P.; Rossmeisl, M.; Bryhn, M.; Kopecky, J. Cellular and molecular effects of n−3 polyunsaturated fatty acids on adipose tissue biology and metabolism. *Clin. Sci.* **2005**, *116*, 1–16. [CrossRef]
10. Namiki, M. Nutraceutical functions of sesame: A review. *Crit. Rev. Food Sci. Nutr.* **2007**, *47*, 651–673. [CrossRef]
11. Whelan, J.; Rust, C. Innovative dietary sources of n-3 fatty acids. *Ann. Rev. Nutr.* **2006**, *26*, 75–103. [CrossRef]
12. Kirby, N.A.; Hester, S.L.; Rees, C.A.; Kennis, R.A.; Zoran, D.L.; Bauer, J.E. Skin surface lipids and skin and hair coat condition in dogs fed increased total fat diets containing polyunstaurated fatty acids. *J. Anim. Physiol. Anim. Nutr.* **2009**, *93*, 505–511. [CrossRef] [PubMed]
13. Blaskovic, M.; Rosenkrantz, W.; Neuber, A.; Sauter-Louis, C.; Mueller, R.S. The effect of a spot- on formulation containing polyunsaturated fatty acids and essential oils on dogs with atopic dermatitis. *Vet. J.* **2014**, *199*, 39–43. [CrossRef] [PubMed]
14. Johnson, L.N.; Heinze, C.R.; Linder, D.E.; Freeman, L.M. Evaluation of marketing claims, ingredients and nutrient profiles of over-the-counter diets market for skin and coat health of dogs. *J. Am. Vet. Med. Assoc.* **2015**, *246*, 1334–1339. [CrossRef] [PubMed]
15. Jamroz, D. *Żywienie Zwierząt i Paszoznawstwo. Tom 3. Paszoznawstwo*; PWN: Warszawa, Poland, 2015; pp. 245–246.
16. Barabasz, B.; Bieniek, J. *Króliki. Towarowa Produkcja Mięsna*; PWRiL: Warszawa, Polska, 2003; pp. 16–32.
17. AOAC International. *Official Methods of Analysis of AOAC*, 18th ed.; 4th Revision; AOAC International: Gaithersburg, MD, USA, 2011.
18. Gugołek, A.; Bielański, P.; Kowalska, D.; Świątkiewicz, S.; Zoń, A. *Zalecenia Żywieniowe i Wartość Pokarmowa Pasz. Zwierzęta Futerkowe*; PAN IFiŻŻ: Jabłonna, Poland, 2011.
19. Sokoła-Wysoczańska, E.; Wysoczański, T.; Czyż, K.; Vogt, A.; Patkowska-Sokoła, B.; Sokoła, K.; Bodkowski, R.; Wyrostek, A.; Roman, K. Charakterystyka estrów etylowych wielonienasyconych kwasów tłuszczowych o wysokiej zawartości kwasu alfa-linolenowego jako składnika biologicznie aktywnych preparatów prozdrowotnych. *Przem. Chem.* **2014**, *93*, 1923–1927.
20. Stark, A.H.; Reifen, R.; Crawford, M. Past and Present Insights on Alpha Linolenic Acid and the Omega-3 Fatty Acid Family. *Crit. Rev. Food* **2016**, *56*, 2261–2267. [CrossRef] [PubMed]
21. Christopherson, S.W.; Glass, R.L. Preparation of milk fat methyl esters by alcohollysis in an essentially non alcoholic. Solution 1. *J. Dairy Sci.* **1969**, *52*, 1289–1290. [CrossRef]
22. Haiqi, G.; Bingjing, L.; Han, L.; Zongcail, Z. Thickness Method for Measuring Hair Density of Rex Rabbit. *Anim. Husb. Feed Sci.* **2018**, *10*, 81–83, 108.
23. Bivainytė, A.; Mikučionienė, D.; Kerpauskas, P. Investigation on thermal properties of double-layered weft knitted fabrics. *Medžiagotyra* **2012**, *18*, 167–171. [CrossRef]
24. Hansen, K.K.; Rode, C.; de Place Hansen, E.J.; Padfield, T.; Kristiansen, F. Experimental Investigation of The Hygrothermal Performance of Insulation Materials. In Proceedings of the DOE/ORNL/ASHRAE/BETEC/ NRC/CIBCE Conference. Performance of Exterior Envelopes of Whole Buildings VIII: Integration of Building Envelopes, Clearwater Beach, FL, USA, 2–7 December 2001; p. 10.
25. Żyliński, T. *Metrologia Włókiennicza. Tom IV*; WNT: Warszawa, Poland, 1973.
26. Bucişcanu, I.I. Sustainable alternatives for wool valorization. *Ann. Univ. Oradea Fasc. Textile Leatherwork* **2014**, *2*, 27–32.
27. Ye, Z.; Wells, C.M.; Carrington, G.C.; Hewitt, N.J. Thermal conductivity of wool and wool hemp insulation. *Int. J. Energy Res.* **2006**, *30*, 37–49. [CrossRef]
28. Oğulata, R.T. The effect of thermal insulation of clothing on human thermal comfort. *Fibres Text. East. Eur.* **2007**, *61*, 67–72.
29. Sirvydas, P.A.; Nadzeikienė, J.; Milašius, R.; Eičinas, J.; Kerpauskas, P. The role of the textile layer in the garment package in suppressing transient heat exchange processes. *Fibres Text. East. Eur.* **2006**, *56*, 55–58.
30. Barauskas, R.; Valasevičiūtė, L.; Jurevičiūtė, A. Computational analysis and experimental investigation of heat and moisture transfer in multilayer textile package. *Medžiagotyra* **2009**, *15*, 80–85.
31. Baron, P.A. Measurment of fibres. In *NIOSH Manual of Analytical Methods (NMAM™)*; US NIOSH: Cincinnati, OH, USA, 2003; pp. 143–161.

32. McGregor, B.A.; Butler, K.L.; Ferguson, M.B. Variation in mohair staple length over the lifetime of Angora goats. *Anim. Prod. Sci.* **2012**, *53*, 479–486. [CrossRef]
33. Kowalski, K.; Włodarczyk, B.; Kowalski, T.M. Probabilistic model of dynamic forces in thread in the knitting zone of weft knitting machines, allowing for the heterogeneity of visco-elasticity yarn properties. *Fibres Text. East. Eur.* **2010**, *18*, 61–67.
34. Mustata, A. Mechanical behaviour in the wet and dry stage of romanian yarns made from flax and hemp. *Fibres Text. East. Eur.* **2010**, *18*, 7–12.
35. Qiu, H.; Quiao, G.M. Evaluation of the significance of processing parameters for the characteristics of interlaced yarn. *Fibres Text. East. Eur.* **2010**, *18*, 26–28. [CrossRef]
36. Khalil, M.H.; Ibrahim, M.K.; El-Deghadi, A.S. Genetic evaluation of fru traits in New Zealand white and Californian rabbits raised on high ambient temperature. *World Rabbit Sci.* **1998**, *6*, 311–318.
37. Taha, E.A.; Samia, A.H.; Nasr, A.I. Evaluating skin quality of some rabbit breeds under egyptian conditions. *World Rabbit Sci.* **2017**, *25*, 193–200. [CrossRef]
38. Rafat, S.A.; de Rochambeau, H.; Brims, M.; Thébault, R.G.; Deretz, S.; Bonnet, M.; Allain, D. Characteristics of Angora rabbit fiber using optical fiber diameter analyzer. *J. Anim. Sci.* **2007**, *85*, 3116–3122. [CrossRef]
39. Mengüç, G.S.; Özdil, N.; Kayseri, G.O. Physical properties of Angora rabbit fibers. *Am. J. Mater. Sci.* **2014**, *2*, 11–13.
40. Onal, L.; Korkmaz, M.; Tutak, M. Relations between the Characteristics of Angora Rabbit Fibre. *Fibers Polym.* **2007**, *8*, 198–204. [CrossRef]
41. Beroual, K.; Maameri, Z.; Halmi, S.; Benleksira, B.; Agabou, A.; Hamdi Pacha, Y. Effects of *Linum usitatissimum* L. ingestion and oil topical application on hair growth in rabbit. *Int. J. Med. Arom. Plants* **2013**, *3*, 459–463.
42. Wyrostek, A.; Roman, K.; Czyż, K.; Janczak, M.; Patkowska-Sokoła, B. Analiza okrywy włosowej kotów domowych ze szczególnym uwzględnieniem budowy histologicznej. *Rocz. Nauk. Pol. Tow. Zootech.* **2017**, *13*, 47–58.
43. Roman, K.; Wyrostek, A.; Czyż, K.; Janczak, M.; Patkowska-Sokoła, B. Charakterystyka okrywy włosowej konika polskiego i konia huculskiego z uwzględnieniem właściwości fizycznych oraz budowy histologicznej różnych rodzajów włosów. *Rocz. Nauk. Pol. Tow. Zootech.* **2016**, *12*, 95–104.
44. Jankowska, D.; Janczak, H.; Bodkowski, R.; Sadkowska, E. Analiza okrywy włosowej psów rasy collie rough z uwzględnieniem jej właściwości przędnych. *Zesz. Nauk. UP Wrocław LVII* **2008**, *567*, 101–108.
45. Przysiecki, P.; Filistowicz, A.; Gorajewska, E.; Filistowicz, A.; Nawrocki, Z.; Nowicki, S. The effect of genotype on coat traits in Arctic foxes during summer and winter season. *J. Agrobiol.* **2009**, *26*, 45–49.
46. Fatahi, I.I.; Alamdar Yazdi, A. Assessment of the relationship between air permeability of woven fabrics and its mechanical properties. *Fibres Text. East. Eur.* **2010**, *18*, 68–71.
47. Ragaišiene, A.; Rusinavičiūte, J. Comparitive investigation of mechanical indices of sheep's wool and dog hair fibre. *Fibres Text. East. Eur.* **2012**, *20*, 43–47.
48. Truter, E.V. *Introduction to Natural Protein Fibres*; Basic Chemistry Fibres Science Series; Paul Elek Scientific Books Ltd.: London, UK, 1973.
49. Sahajpal, V.; Goyal, S.P.; Jayapal, R.; Yoganand, K.; Thakar, M.K. Hair characteristics of four Indian bear species. *Sci. Justice* **2008**, *48*, 8–15. [CrossRef]
50. Kamalakannan, M.; De, J.K. Hair Morphology of Striped Hyena Hyaena hyaena (Linnaeus, 1758). *Int. J. Curr. Microbiol. Appl. Sci.* **2017**, *6*, 1438–1441. [CrossRef]
51. Zhang, Y.; Zheng, Q.T.; Wang, X.Q.; Liu, H.W. Structure Structural Characteristics of Rabbit Hair. *Adv. Mat. Res.* **2011**, *332–334*, 1073–1076. [CrossRef]
52. Zheng, Q.T.; Zhang, Y.; Yang, M.X.; Liu, H.W. Morphological Structures of Rabbit Hair. *Adv. Mat. Res.* **2011**, *332–334*, 1063–1066. [CrossRef]
53. Momota, Y.; Shimada, K.; Kadoya, C.; Gin, A.; Kobayashi, J.; Nakamura, Y.; Matsubara, T.; Sako, T. The effect of a herbal paste and oil extract on the lipid content of canine hair fibres. *Vet. Dermatol.* **2017**, *28*, e337–e373. [CrossRef]
54. Sinclair, A.J.; Attar-Bashi, N.M.; Li, D. What is the role of α-linolenic acid for mammals? *Lipids* **2002**, *37*, 1113–1123. [CrossRef]
55. Cerrato, S.; Ramió-Lluch, L.; Fondevila, D.; Rodes, D.; Brazis, P.; Puigdemont, A. Effects of Essential Oils and Polyunsaturated Fatty Acids on Canine Skin Equivalents: Skin Lipid Assessment and Morphological Evaluation. *J. Vet. Med.* **2013**, *2013*, 1–9. [CrossRef]
56. Jhala, A.J.; Hall, L.M. Flax (*Linum usitatissimum* L.): Current uses and future applications. *Aust. J. Basic Appl. Sci.* **2010**, *4*, 4304–4312.
57. Burdge, G.C.; Calder, P.C. Conversion of alpha-linolenic acid to longer chain polyunsaturated fatty acids in human adults. *Reprod. Nutr. Dev.* **2005**, *45*, 581–597. [CrossRef]
58. Tres, A.; Bou, R.; Codony, C.; Guardiola, F. Dietary n-6- or n-3-rich vegetable fats and a-tocopheryl acetate: Effects on fatty acid composition and stability of rabbit plasma, liver and meat. *Animal* **2009**, *3*, 1408–1419. [CrossRef]
59. Cherian, G.; Sim, J.S. Dietary alpha-linolenic acid alters the fatty acid composition of lipid classes in swine tissues. *J. Agric. Food Chem.* **1995**, *43*, 2911–2916. [CrossRef]
60. D'Arrigo, M.; Hoz, L.; Lopez-Bote, C.J.; Cambero, M.I.; Pin, C.; Ordonez, J.A. Effect of dietary linseed oil on pig hepatic tissue fatty acid composition and susceptibility to lipid peroxidation. *Nutr. Res.* **2002**, *22*, 1189–1196. [CrossRef]

61. Hoz, L.; Lopez-Bote, C.J.; Cambero, M.I.; D'Arrigo, M.; Pin, C.; Santos, C.; Ordonez, J.A. Effect of dietary linseed oil and alpha-tocopherol on pork tenderloin (psoas major) muscle. *Meat Sci.* **2003**, *65*, 1039–1044. [CrossRef]
62. Nuernberg, K.; Fischer, K.; Nuernberg, G.; Küchenmeister, U.; Klosowska, D.; Eliminowska-Wenda, G.; Fiedler, I.; Eder, K. Effects of dietary olive and linseed oil on lipid composition, meat quality, sensory characteristics and muscle structure in pigs. *Meat Sci.* **2005**, *70*, 63–74. [CrossRef]
63. Arterburn, L.M.; Hall, E.B.; Oken, H. Distribution, interconversion, and dose response of n-3 fatty acids in humans. *Am. J. Clin. Nutr.* **2006**, *83*, 1467S–1476S. [CrossRef] [PubMed]
64. Bernardini, M.; Dal Bosco, A.; Castellini, C. Effect of dietary n-3/n-6 ratio on fatty acid composition of liver, meat and perirenal fat in rabbits. *Animal Sci.* **1999**, *68*, 647–654. [CrossRef]
65. Dal Bosco, A.; Castellini, C.; Bianchi, L.; Mugnai, C. Effect of dietary alinolenic acid and vitamin E on the fatty acid composition, storage stability and sensory traits of rabbit meat. *Meat Sci.* **2004**, *66*, 407–413. [CrossRef]
66. Enser, M.; Richardson, R.I.; Wood, J.D.; Gill, B.P.; Sheard, P.R. Feeding linseed to increase the n-3 PUFA of pork: Fatty acid composition of muscle, adipose tissue, liver and sausages. *Meat Sci.* **2000**, *55*, 201–212. [CrossRef]
67. Rafay, J.; Parkányi, V. The rabbit as a model and farm animal at the research Institute for animal production nitra: A review. *Slovak J. Anim. Sci.* **2016**, *49*, 141–146.

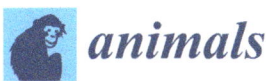

Article

# Effect of Dietary Rosemary and Ginger Essential Oils on the Growth Performance, Feed Utilization, Meat Nutritive Value, Blood Biochemicals, and Redox Status of Growing NZW Rabbits

Mahmoud A. Elazab [1], Ayman M. Khalifah [1], Abdelmotaleb A. Elokil [2], Alaa E. Elkomy [1,3], Marwa M. Rabie [4], Abdallah Tageldein Mansour [5,6] and Sabrin Abdelrahman Morshedy [6,*]

[1] Livestock Research Department, Arid Lands Cultivation Research Institute, City of Scientific Research and Technological Applications, Alexandria 21934, Egypt; melazab@srtacity.sci.eg (M.A.E.); akhalifah@srtacity.sci.eg (A.M.K.); alaa_elkomy@yahoo.com (A.E.E.)
[2] Department of Animal Production, Faculty of Agriculture, Benha University, Moshtohor 13736, Egypt; abdelmotaleb@fagr.bu.edu.eg
[3] Faculty of Desert and Environmental Agriculture, Matrouh University, Matrouh 51512, Egypt
[4] Department of Poultry Production, Faculty of Agriculture, Mansoura University, Mansoura 35516, Egypt; m_rabie2009@mans.edu.eg
[5] Animal and Fish Production Department, College of Agricultural and Food Sciences, King Faisal University, Al-Ahsa 31982, Saudi Arabia; amansour@kfu.edu.sa
[6] Fish and Animal Production Department, Faculty of Agriculture (Saba Basha), Alexandria University, Alexandria 21531, Egypt
* Correspondence: sabrin_morshedy@alexu.edu.eg

**Citation:** Elazab, M.A.; Khalifah, A.M.; Elokil, A.A.; Elkomy, A.E.; Rabie, M.M.; Mansour, A.T.; Morshedy, S.A. Effect of Dietary Rosemary and Ginger Essential Oils on the Growth Performance, Feed Utilization, Meat Nutritive Value, Blood Biochemicals, and Redox Status of Growing NZW Rabbits. Animals 2022, 12, 375. https://doi.org/10.3390/ani12030375

Academic Editors: Iveta Plachá, Monika Pogány Simonová, Andrea Lauková and Juan José Pascual

Received: 10 December 2021
Accepted: 27 January 2022
Published: 3 February 2022

**Publisher's Note:** MDPI stays neutral with regard to jurisdictional claims in published maps and institutional affiliations.

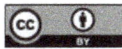

**Copyright:** © 2022 by the authors. Licensee MDPI, Basel, Switzerland. This article is an open access article distributed under the terms and conditions of the Creative Commons Attribution (CC BY) license (https:// creativecommons.org/licenses/by/ 4.0/).

**Simple Summary:** The rabbit farming industry has gained more interest due to its high productivity, high growth rate, and high-quality meat. One of the public health concerns is that global rabbit production is expected to increase to meet the increasing demand for lean meat. In the present study, we focused on the use of phytogenic feed additives (essential oils of rosemary (REO) and ginger (GEO)) as environmentally friendly supplementation to improve rabbit growth performance, physiological status, and meat quality. The results indicated that the use of REO and GEO at a dose of 0.5% dramatically improved the growth performance and feed utilization of treated rabbits. The cholesterol level decreased significantly in rabbit plasma and meat after REO and GEO treatments. The fat content tended to decline in the muscles and the triglycerides were remarkedly reduced in the plasma of treated animals. In addition, the oxidant/antioxidant balance in the plasma could be improved with supplementation with a high dose of REO and GEO. Accordingly, the use of REO and GEO as supplementations for growing rabbits could contribute to improving the sustainable production of the rabbit industry.

**Abstract:** This study was conducted to assess the impacts of using two essential oils, rosemary and ginger, on growing rabbits' performance, carcass traits, meat composition, blood biochemicals, and the redox status of growing New Zealand White (NZW) rabbits. A total of 120 unsexed NZW rabbits, 42-days-old, were assigned randomly to five experimental groups ($n = 24$, 6 replicates with 4 rabbits each). The first group received a basal diet (control), the second to fifth groups were dietary supplemented daily with rosemary essential oil (REO) and ginger essential oil (GEO) at doses of 0.25 and 0.5% for each supplementation (REO-0.25, REO-0.5, GEO-0.25, and GEO-0.5), respectively. The growth traits were studied for 7 weeks, from the 7th to the 13th week of the rabbits' age. The results revealed that final body weight, weight gain, and average daily gain increased significantly ($p < 0.01$) in the REO-0.5 and GEO-0.5 treatments compared to the control group. Daily feed intake decreased ($p = 0.005$) in essential oil treatments. Meanwhile, the feed conversion ratio improved significantly ($p = 0.001$) in REO and GEO at the high doses compared to the control group. The weight percentages of liver and giblets increased ($p < 0.001$) with both treatments of REO and GEO compared to the control group. The dietary supplementation with REO and GEO did not affect ($p > 0.05$) the meat composition of *Longissimus dorsi* and hind leg muscles. Meanwhile, REO and GEO supplementation significantly decreased cholesterol levels in the rabbit meat. Thiobarbituric acid reactive substance concentrations decreased by 10 and 15% in the meat of REO-0.5 and GEO-0.5 treatments, respectively, compared to the other groups. In the same trend, REO and GEO treatments induced a significant ($p = 0.001$) reduction in the plasma cholesterol concentrations and triglycerides compared to the control. The total antioxidant capacity increased by 7.60% and the malondialdehyde decreased by 11.64% in the plasma of GEO-0.5 treatment than the control. Thus, the dietary supplementation of REO and GEO have a beneficial effect in improving the productivity and meat quality of growing rabbits.

**Keywords:** rabbit meat quality; rosemary essential oil; ginger essential oil; growth performance; lipid profile; antioxidant balance

## 1. Introduction

Rabbit meat has undoubtedly been a component of human nutrition for a long time. Moreover, the world's consumption of rabbit meat grows year on year due to its good taste, special flavor, and diverse uses in preparing a wide variety of foods [1,2]. Commonly, rabbit meat is consumed in Egypt and several Mediterranean countries. [3,4]. Furthermore, rabbit meat is especially beneficial in Western countries, where people's diets are often high in lipids and salt, putting them at risk of obesity, cardiovascular disease, and hypertension [3].

Recently, the rabbit industry has gained much more interest due to the fact that rabbit meat has several benefits, which qualify it to become one of the most promising healthy foods [5]. Rabbit meat is an excellent source of nutrients, including proteins, B vitamins, and minerals [4]. The functional proteins in rabbit meat have been recognized as one of the highest quality proteins in digestibility, as well as amino acid composition. Furthermore, rabbit meat is free of uric acid and has a low purine level [1,2]. In addition, rabbit meats have lower contents of salt, fat, cholesterol (59 mg/100 g of muscle) and have a lower energy value (789 kJ/100 g meat) than other species' meat [6,7]. Furthermore, the majority of their energy comes from proteins [4]. The fatty acid composition of rabbit meat is characterized by a high polyunsaturated fatty acids (PUFA) content, especially omega-3, PUFA, which plays an important function in human nutrition by assisting in the prevention of lifestyle diseases [8,9].

The different production factors, especially feeding, have a strong influence on growth performance, reproduction, and product quality [10], as well as the chemical composition of rabbit meat, particularly regarding fat content [2]. For this reason, natural sources of feed additives can be used as a significant tool in rabbit nutrition for improving growth, feed efficiency, and reproduction, as well as lowering disease incidence and the house emissions of rabbits [11–13]. There is a significant motivation for phytogenic feed additives as a potential alternative to using synthetic antibiotics as growth promoters since the European Union banned growth promoters in 2006. In addition, the regulations are being tightened in the United States [14–16]. This ban is due to safety concerns about bacterial resistance to the synthesized antibiotics and the hazardous residuals in meat, milk, and eggs, which would pose a great threat to human health [17,18].

In this regard, probiotics, organic acids, exogenous enzymes, propolis, and plant secondary compounds, such as saponins, tannins, and essential oils (EOs) have all been recommended as natural alternatives [16]. Aromatic plants contain EOs, which can be used as phytogenic feed additives, these oils are characterized as volatile, odorous, hydrophobic, and highly concentrated compounds [19]. Essential oils are aromatic oily liquids extracted by distillation from various plant components such as flowers, buds, seeds, leaves, twigs, bark, wood, fruits, and roots [20–22].

Among all herbs and spices, rosemary (*Rosmarinus officinalis* L.) could be considered to contain the highest level of biologically active compounds [23]. Rosemary extracts, which are primarily made from dried rosemary leaves, are popular in feed additives and the pharmaceutical business because they have numerous health benefits, including antioxidant, antibacterial, anti-inflammatory, and anticancer properties as well as cognitive-enhancing potential [24]. The essential oil of rosemary (REO) contains several compounds at different concentrations.

Ginger from the Zingiberaceae family (*Zingiber officinale*) has long been used as a spice and herbal remedy. There are several terpene components in ginger essential oil, such as β-bisabolene, α-curcumene, zingiberene, α-farnesene, and β-sesquiphellandrene [25,26]. Ginger has pharmacological properties that manage and prevent gastrointestinal disorders, neurodegenerative diseases, atherosclerosis, cardiovascular complications, liver and kidney failure, diabetes, metabolic syndrome, cancer, and emesis/nausea [27]. In addition, ginger's constituents participate in biological processes, such as apoptosis, DNA deterioration, chromatin and epigenetic regulation, regulation of cytoskeletal and adhesion, immunology and inflammation, and neuroscience [25,28].

Diets containing rosemary or ginger root significantly improved the growth performance of growing rabbits [3,29,30]. Moreover, feeding diets enriched with EOs significantly affected the carcass traits of rabbits [3,5]. Several studies found that EOs decreased both cholesterol and triglyceride levels [31–34]. Thus improving the oxidative stability and effectively delaying the lipid oxidation of rabbit meat by the dietary supplementation of rosemary aqueous extracts [3] or ginger powder [35].

Essential oils have been shown to improve the synthesis of digestive secretions and nutrient absorption in animals, as well as lower pathogenic stress in the gut, exert antioxidant characteristics, and strengthen the immune system, which helps to explain the observed improvement in their performance [36,37]. It is hypothesized that the dietary addition of rosemary essential oil (REO) and ginger essential oil (GEO) is expected to exert beneficial effects on growth performance, feed utilization, blood biochemicals, antioxidant status, carcass traits, and meat quality of growing rabbits. Therefore, the current study was designed to evaluate the effect of the dietary inclusion of two levels of REO and GEO (0.25 and 0.5%) in four experimental treatments on the performance, blood biochemicals, and meat quality of NZW growing rabbits.

## 2. Materials and Methods

### 2.1. Ethics Approval and Consent to Participate

Rabbits were handled in the present study following the guidelines of the Pharmaceutical & Fermentation Industries Development Center, City of Scientific Research and Technology Applications, (SRTA-City), Alexandria, Egypt, after the approval of the Institutional Animal Care and Use Committees (IACUCs)/IACUC # 37-6F-1021.

### 2.2. Animals, Experimental Design, and Housing Environment

A total of 120 unsexed NZW rabbits, aged 6 weeks, with an average body weight of 850 ± 50 g were used in this experiment. Rabbits were divided randomly into five groups ($n$ = 24, 6 replicates in each group with 4 rabbits in each replicate). The 1st group received a basal diet (control). The 2nd to 5th groups were dietary supplemented daily with rosemary essential oil (REO) and ginger essential oil (GEO) at doses of 0.25 and 0.5% for each supplement (REO-0.25, REO-0.5, GEO-0.25, and GEO-0.5), respectively. The essential oils were weighed daily for each dose and added to the half amount of the ration and mixed well with pelleted basal diet to ensure the consumption of the actual dose of EOs and avoiding the loss of EOs with uneaten feed or auto-oxidation. In addition, to avoid the effect of the solvent (oil) of the essential oils, corn oil was supplemented to the basal diet of the control at a level of 0.25%. The next portion was added after the complete intake of the first portion. The experimental treatments lasted 7 weeks from the 7th to the 13th week of the rabbits' age.

The present study was conducted at a private farm located in Borg El-Arab city, Alexandria Governorate, Egypt during February and March 2020. A total of 4 rabbits in each replicate were housed in a galvanized wire cage (dimensions: 60 cm × 40 cm × 30 cm) with a feeder and an automatic nipple drinker. All rabbits were kept under similar management, hygienic and environmental conditions throughout the experimental period. The average ambient temperature was 18–23 °C and the daily photoperiod was a 16:8 h light-dark cycle with a semi-continuous lighting program. The basal experimental diet was formulated and pelleted to meet the nutrient requirements of rabbits, according to NRC [38]. The ingredients of the basal experimental diet are shown in Table 1. The composition of the basal diet (Table 1) was calculated according to Villamide, et al. [39]. The pelleted diets and freshwater were provided ad libitum.

**Table 1.** The ingredients and calculated chemical composition of the experimental diet.

| Ingredients | (g/kg) | Calculated Chemical Composition | (g/kg as Fed Basis) |
|---|---|---|---|
| Lucerne hay | 365 | Crude protein (CP) | 177.2 |
| Ground barley grains | 160 | Ether extract (EE) | 24.6 |
| Ground yellow corn | 120 | Crude fiber (CF) | 127.6 |
| Wheat barn | 180 | Calcium (Ca) | 10.6 |
| Soybean meal (44% CP) | 130 | Total phosphorus (P) | 3.8 |
| Common Salt (NaCl) | 5 | Lysine | 9.1 |
| Beet molasses | 20 | Methionine | 4.3 |
| Dicalcium phosphate | 5 | Methionine + Cystine | 7.7 |
| Ground limestone | 10 | Digestible energy (DE), kcal/kg | 2574 |
| Vit. & Min. Premix [1] | 2 | | |
| DL-Methionine | 2 | | |
| Anti-toxicants | 1 | | |

[1] Each kg contains: Vit. A, 20,000 IU; Vit. E, 8.33 g; Vit. D$_3$, 15,000 IU; Vit. K, 0.33 g; Vit. B$_1$, 1.0 g; Vit. B$_2$, 1.0 g; Vit. B$_6$, 0.33 g; Vit. B$_{12}$, 1.7 mg; Vit. B$_5$, 8.33 g; Pantothenic acid, 3.33 g; Niacin, 8.33 g; Folic acid, 0.83 g; Biotin, 33 mg; Choline chloride, 20 g; Zn, 11.7 g; Fe, 12.5 g; Cu, 0.5 g; Co, 1.33 mg; Se, 16.6 mg; Mn, 5 g and antioxidants, 10 g.

*2.3. Chemical Analysis for Active Components of Rosemary and Ginger Essential Oils*

The individual essential oils (EOs) of rosemary (*Rosmarinus officinalis* L.) and ginger (*Zingiber Officinalis*) were produced by the El-Hawag Factory for the extraction of Natural Oils and Cosmetics in Badr City, Egypt. The volatile contents of the oils were determined by the gas chromatography-mass spectrometry technique (GC-MS) (Table 2). The analysis of GC-MS was carried out using a Shimadzu capillary gas chromatographic system directly attached to the mass spectrometer (GC-MS–model QP 2010; (Shimadzu) DB–5 ms non-polar fused silica capillary column (30 m × 0.25 mm, 0.25 m film thickness) under the following conditions: oven temperature increased with a rate of 3 °C/min from 70 to 200 °C, and then maintained for 35 min, injection temperature: 200 °C, injection volume: 1 µL, split ratio: 100:1, carrier gas: helium, gas flow rate: 1.51 mL/min, linear velocity: 45.1 cm/s, Mass spectra were obtained at 70 eV of ionization energy, ionization source temperature: 200 °C.

**Table 2.** List of the active components profile of rosemary and ginger essential oils.

| Component Identified | Area (%) |
|---|---|
| Rosemary Essential Oil (REO, *Rosmarinus officinalis*) | |
| Limonene | 23.03 |
| Cis- Vaccenic acid | 12.91 |
| Trans-4- Decadienal | 10.67 |
| Octane, 2, 4, 6- trimethyl | 9.14 |
| 9, 12 Octadecadienoic acid | 8.77 |
| Trans-3-Nonene | 7.65 |
| 4-Heptenal | 6.9 |
| Eucalyptol | 3.98 |
| Linalool | 3.5 |
| 2-Decenal | 2.96 |
| 2-Undecenal | 2.49 |
| Octadecanoic acid | 1.61 |
| Unidentified peaks | 6.39 |
| Ginger essential oil (GEO, *Zingiber Officinalis*) | |
| Zingiberene | 29.74 |
| Carveol | 15.05 |
| Cyclohexene.3-(1, 5-dimethyl-4-hexenyl)-6-methylene | 10.4 |
| 9, 12 Octadecadienoic acid | 9.2 |
| Cis-alpha- Bisabolene | 5.04 |
| *n*-Hexadecanoic acid | 3.93 |
| Alpha- Farnesene | 2.88 |
| Unidentified peaks | 23.76 |

## 2.4. Growth Performance Measurements

Rabbits were individually weighed in the morning before offering the feed. The initial and final body weights (BW) were recorded using a digital balance. The body weight gain (BWG) was calculated as the difference between final and initial BW and the average daily gain (ADG) was calculated as BWG divided by the number of days of the experimental period (49 days). Daily feed intake (FI) was recorded for each replicate throughout the whole experimental period, as the difference between the offered and refused feed. The feed conversion (FCR) ratio was calculated by dividing average daily feed intake/average daily gain.

## 2.5. Carcass Traits and Meat Composition

At the end of the experiment, six rabbits per treatment were randomly chosen for carcass evaluations. The rabbits were weighed pre-slaughter after fasting for 12 h then slaughtered by cutting the carotid artery and jugular vein for complete depletion. Just after bleeding, carcasses were skinned and eviscerated. The hot eviscerated carcass with a head, giblets (liver, heart, kidneys), and spleen were weighed. The carcass yields were determined as a proportion of the rabbits' pre-slaughter live body weight. Additionally, the following equations are the percentages of total edible components, non-edible portions, and giblets:

$$\text{Giblets\%} = \text{kidney\%} + \text{heart\%} + \text{liver\%}. \tag{1}$$

$$\text{Total edible parts\%} = \text{hot carcass\%} + \text{Giblets\%}. \tag{2}$$

$$\text{Non-edible parts\%} = 100 - \text{total edible parts\%}. \tag{3}$$

The carcass was chilled for 24 h at 3 °C to evaluate the quality of rabbit meat. The chilled carcass was then dissected and their *Longissimus dorsi* (LD) and hind leg (HL) muscles were excised according to the recommended procedures of the World Rabbit Science Association [40]. The samples of LD and HL were individually vacuum packaged and stored at −20 °C until analyses. Meat samples were chemically analyzed for the moisture, crude protein, ether extract, and ash contents according to AOAC [41]. The cholesterol content of meat samples was determined according to the procedure described by Dinh, et al. [42]. The lipid oxidation status of LD samples was measured using the thiobarbituric acid reactive substances (TBARS) method and its products were expressed as malondialdehyde (MDA) equivalents (mg MDA/kg muscle) according to the method of Dal Bosco, et al. [43].

## 2.6. Plasma Biochemical and Antioxidant Status

Six blood samples from each treatment were obtained concurrently at slaughter in heparinized test tubes, centrifuged for separating plasma, and frozen at −20 °C for further examination. The plasma concentration of triglycerides, total cholesterol, and high-density lipoprotein-cholesterol (HDL-c) and low-density lipoprotein-cholesterol (LDL-c) were estimated colorimetrically by using commercial kits produced by (Biodiagnostic® kit, Egypt). In addition, total antioxidant capacity (TAC) and MDA concentrations were measured colorimetrically according to Koracevic, et al. [44] and Banjare, et al. [45], respectively.

## 2.7. Statistical Analysis

The effect of EOs on the measured variables was analyzed statistically by one-way analysis of variance (ANOVA) using a completely randomized design. The statistical analysis was conducted using SPSS11.0 statistical software. The statistical model was used as follows:

$$x_{ij} = \mu + T_i + e_{ij},$$

where $x_{ij}$ is the value of the measured variable, $\mu$ is the overall mean, $T_i$ is the effect of treatment (i = 5 treatments), and $e_{ij}$ is the residual error. Duncan's multiple range test [46] was used to compare treatment means wherever significant differences were detected at a *p*-value equal to or less than 0.05 for normally distributed data, for the non-normally distributed data, James—Howell was used as a post hoc measure for multiple comparisons. The percentage data were transformed to arc sign before the analysis [47], but the data were presented as a percentage.

## 3. Results

### 3.1. Growth Performance of Growing Rabbits

The results of growth performance of the growing NZW rabbits as affected by the dietary inclusion of REO and GEO from 7th to 13th weeks of age are shown in Table 3. The results showed that FBW, BWG, and ADG significantly increased ($p < 0.001$) in REO-0.5 and GEO-0.5 groups compared to the control group. Daily feed intake of rabbits that received REO and GEO at the highest dose were significantly lower ($p = 0.005$) than other groups. The dietary supplementation with REO and GEO at the highest doses improved ($p = 0.001$) FCR compared to the control group.

**Table 3.** Effect of the dietary supplementation of rosemary and ginger essential oils on the growth performance of the growing NZW rabbits from 7th to 13th week of age ($n = 24$, 6 replicates in each group with 4 rabbits in each replicate).

| Items | Control | REO-0.25 | REO-0.5 | GEO-0.25 | GEO-0.5 | SEM | *p*-Value |
|---|---|---|---|---|---|---|---|
| Initial body weight, g | 853.4 | 850.1 | 849.5 | 848.4 | 853.1 | 2.16 | 0.543 |
| Final body weight, g | 1965 [b] | 1997 [ab] | 2068 [a] | 2000 [ab] | 2075 [a] | 20.22 | 0.001 |
| Body weight gain, g | 1112 [b] | 1147 [b] | 1218 [a] | 1152 [b] | 1222 [a] | 18.64 | 0.001 |
| Average daily gain, g | 22.69 [b] | 23.41 [b] | 24.86 [a] | 23.50 [b] | 24.93 [a] | 0.38 | 0.001 |
| Daily feed intake, g | 82.09 [a] | 81.25 [ab] | 80.21 [b] | 81.65 [a] | 79.85 [b] | 0.31 | 0.005 |
| Feed conversion ratio, g | 3.63 [a] | 3.48 [ab] | 3.22 [b] | 3.48 [ab] | 3.20 [b] | 0.05 | 0.001 |

[a–b]: Means in the same row bearing different superscripts are significantly different ($p \leq 0.05$). REO-0.25 and REO-0.5: rosemary essential oil supplemented with 0.25 and 0.5%, respectively. GEO-0.25 and GEO-0.5: ginger essential oil supplemented with 0.25 and 0.5%, respectively. SEM: standard error of the mean.

### 3.2. Carcass Traits

Table 4 shows the effect of the dietary supplementation of REO and GEO on growing NZW rabbits' carcass traits at the end of the experiment. The dietary supplementation of REO and GEO did not affect ($p > 0.05$) the carcass characteristics of the growing NZW rabbits. The weight percentages of liver and giblets increased ($p < 0.001$) with the dietary supplementation of REO and GEO at different doses compared to the control group.

**Table 4.** Effect of the dietary supplementation of rosemary and ginger essential oils on carcass traits of growing NZW rabbits at the end of the experiment ($n = 6$).

| Items | Control | REO-0.25 | REO-0.5 | GEO-0.25 | GEO-0.5 | SEM | *p*-Value |
|---|---|---|---|---|---|---|---|
| Pre-slaughter live body weight, g | 1978 | 2000 | 2065 | 2011 | 2060 | 6.67 | 0.812 |
| Hot eviscerated carcass with a head, g | 1185 | 1212 | 1254 | 1244 | 1242 | 51.5 | 0.728 |
| Dressed carcass, % | 59.89 | 60.57 | 60.72 | 61.82 | 60.29 | 1.19 | 0.575 |
| Liver, % | 2.22 [c] | 2.40 [b] | 2.46 [ab] | 2.55 [a] | 2.52 [a] | 0.04 | <0.001 |
| Kidneys, % | 0.54 | 0.53 | 0.52 | 0.53 | 0.54 | 0.02 | 0.913 |
| Heart, % | 0.27 | 0.26 | 0.25 | 0.26 | 0.27 | 0.01 | 0.650 |
| Spleen, % | 0.06 | 0.05 | 0.06 | 0.05 | 0.06 | 0.01 | 0.908 |
| Head, % | 4.93 | 4.87 | 4.81 | 4.88 | 4.97 | 0.13 | 0.810 |
| Giblets, % | 3.02 [c] | 3.19 [b] | 3.23 [ab] | 3.34 [a] | 3.32 [a] | 0.03 | <0.001 |
| Total edible parts, % | 62.91 | 63.75 | 64.69 | 65.16 | 65.26 | 0.45 | 0.439 |
| Non-edible parts, % | 37.09 | 36.25 | 35.31 | 34.84 | 34.74 | 0.45 | 0.439 |

[a–c]: Means in the same row bearing different superscripts are significantly different ($p \leq 0.05$). REO-0.25 and REO-0.5: rosemary essential oil supplemented with 0.25 and 0.5%, respectively. GEO-0.25 and GEO-0.5: ginger essential oil supplemented with 0.25 and 0.5%, respectively. SEM: standard error of the mean.

### 3.3. Meat Composition

Table 5 illustrates the effect of the dietary supplementation of REO and GEO on the composition of LD and HL muscles of the growing NZW rabbits at the end of the experiment. There were no significant differences ($p > 0.05$) among treatments on the meat composition of LD and HL muscles. Meanwhile, TBAR's concentration tended to decrease with increasing the supplementation of REO and GEO at the highest doses compared to the other groups. The cholesterol concentration in LD muscles decreased ($p < 0.05$) with the dietary supplementation of REO and GEO at a high level compared to the control group. In the same trend, the cholesterol concentration in the HL muscles decreased ($p < 0.05$) with the dietary supplementation of REO and GEO at both levels compared to the control group.

**Table 5.** Effect of the dietary supplementation of rosemary and ginger essential oils on meat composition traits of the growing NZW rabbits at the end of the experiment ($n = 6$).

| Items | Control | REO-0.25 | REO-0.5 | GEO-0.25 | GEO-0.5 | SEM | p-Value |
|---|---|---|---|---|---|---|---|
| | | Longissimus dorsi muscle | | | | | |
| Moisture (g/100 g meat) | 73.97 | 74.04 | 73.79 | 74.03 | 73.82 | 0.28 | 0.857 |
| Protein (g/100 g meat) | 24.53 | 24.55 | 24.93 | 24.74 | 24.92 | 0.17 | 0.457 |
| Fat (g/100 g meat) | 0.44 | 0.39 | 0.40 | 0.42 | 0.39 | 0.03 | 0.454 |
| Ash (g/100 g meat) | 1.30 | 1.30 | 1.27 | 1.27 | 1.28 | 0.05 | 0.955 |
| Cholesterol (mg/100 g meat) | 50.51 [a] | 49.51 [ab] | 48.20 [b] | 49.50 [ab] | 48.68 [b] | 0.41 | 0.035 |
| TBARS (mg MDA/kg meat) | 0.20 | 0.19 | 0.18 | 0.20 | 0.17 | 0.01 | 0.145 |
| | | Hind leg muscle | | | | | |
| Moisture (g/100 g meat) | 74.15 | 74.11 | 74.22 | 74.30 | 74.30 | 0.05 | 0.209 |
| Protein (g/100 g meat) | 22.09 | 22.04 | 22.03 | 22.14 | 22.18 | 0.08 | 0.699 |
| Fat (g/100 g meat) | 2.44 | 2.41 | 2.40 | 2.39 | 2.39 | 0.06 | 0.883 |
| Ash (g/100 g meat) | 1.25 | 1.24 | 1.24 | 1.26 | 1.24 | 0.02 | 0.840 |
| Cholesterol (mg/100 g of meat) | 66.06 [a] | 65.50 [ab] | 64.39 [bc] | 64.64 [bc] | 63.48 [c] | 0.18 | 0.003 |

[a,b,c]: Means in the same row bearing different superscripts are significantly different ($p \leq 0.05$). REO-0.25 and REO-0.5: rosemary essential oil supplemented with 0.25 and 0.5%, respectively. GEO-0.25 and GEO-0.5: ginger essential oil supplemented with 0.25 and 0.5%, respectively. TBARS: thiobarbituric acid reactive substances. MDA: malondialdehyde. SEM: standard error of the mean.

### 3.4. Lipids Profile and Oxidant/Antioxidant Balance

The effect of the dietary supplementation of REO and GEO on some blood plasma parameters at the end of the experiment of the NZW rabbits from 7th to 13th weeks of age are summarized in Figure 1. Plasma cholesterol concentration was lower ($p = 0.001$) with REO or GEO treatments than in the control group. Similarly, the REO-0.5 and GEO at both doses significantly reduced ($p = 0.001$) plasma triglyceride as compared to the REO-0.25 and the control groups. However, the dietary supplementation of REO and GEO had no significant effects ($p > 0.05$) on plasma HDL-c, LDL-c levels. The dietary supplementation of GEO at the highest dose tended to improve TAC concentrations in plasma and decrease plasma MDA concentrations.

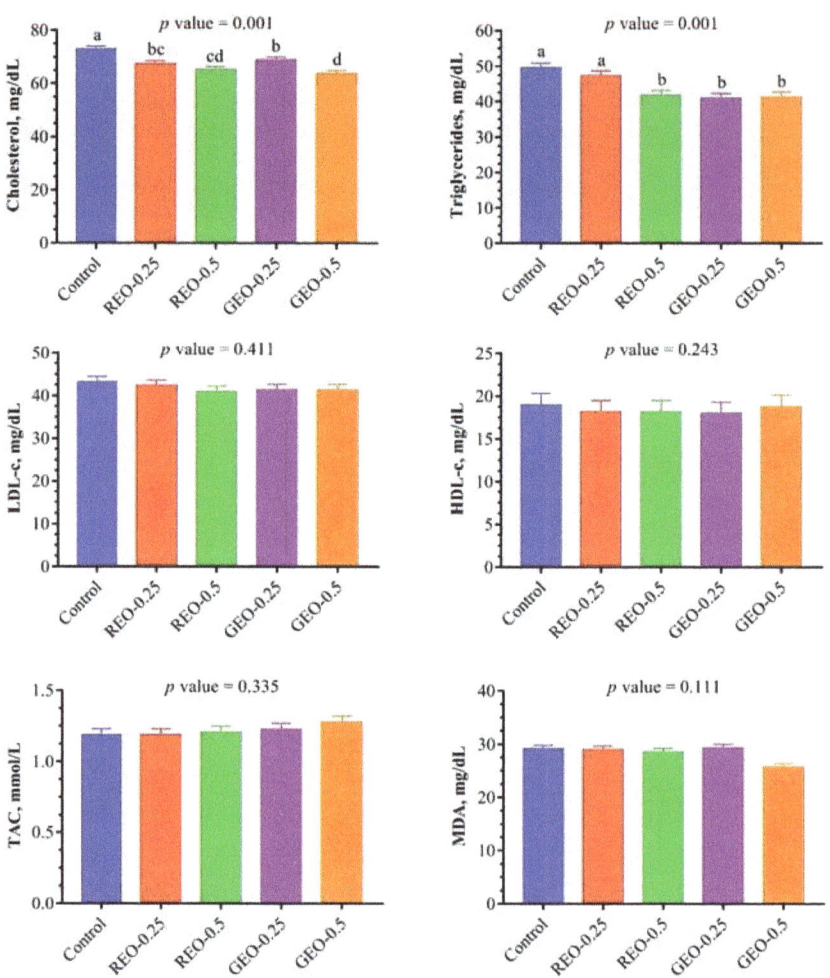

**Figure 1.** Effect of the dietary supplementation of rosemary and ginger essential oils on lipids profile and oxidant/antioxidant balance in plasma of growing NZW rabbits at the end of experiment ($n = 6$, means ± SEM). Bars bearing different superscripts are significantly different ($p \leq 0.05$). REO-0.25 and REO-0.5: rosemary essential oil supplemented with 0.25 and 0.5%, respectively. GEO-0.25 and GEO-0.5: ginger essential oil supplemented with 0.25 and 0.5%, respectively. LDL-c: low-density lipoprotein-cholesterol; HDL-c: high-density lipoprotein-cholesterol; TAC: total antioxidant capacity; MDA: malondialdehyde.

## 4. Discussion

Essential oils exhibit pharmacological properties, such as antibacterial, antimicrobial, antifungal, and antiparasitic properties, which might be due to secondary metabolites found in the oil during processing. Essential oils are low-molecular-weight chemicals that may easily permeate cell membranes and hence participate in metabolic events in the body [48].

In the present study, the dietary supplementation of REO or GEO improved the growth performance of rabbits and the FCR. These improvements could be due to the effect of essential oils on digestion, absorption, and utilization of dietary nutrients [36,37]. In addition, the effects of ginger phytochemicals are exerted by specific signaling pathways linked with the mechanisms and functions of cells, including autophagy, cellular metabolism, mitogen-activated protein kinase, and cell development and differentiation [49]. The present results are consistent with the findings of Cardinali, et al. [3], who found that dietary supplementation with rosemary (0.2%) alone or in combination with oregano extract (0.1% oregano extract + 0.1% rosemary extract) to NZW rabbits had a significant positive effect on FBW and ADG. In addition, diets containing 3% of rosemary powder or 1.5% of ginger root powder significantly improved BWG, WBG, and FCR of NZW rabbits [29]. Additionally, the increasing of ginger powder levels in growing rabbits' diets (1, 2, and 3%) enhanced growth performance and this may be due to improving the appetite and feed utilization [30]. However, in the present study feed intake reduced with the increasing supplementation levels of both essential oils, this may be due to the high concentrations of active molecules in the essential oils in comparison to the dried ginger powder, which could cause an irritating odor and repellent smell of the ration [16]. On the other hand, the growth performance of growing rabbits was not affected by the dietary inclusion of REO at a level of 0.15% [50] or 0.25, 0.5, and 0.75 g/kg of diet [51]. Previous studies have shown that herbal oils can help in improving growth performance by increasing feed intake and/or stimulating the secretion of enzymes, resulting in better nutrient digestion and absorption through the gut [52,53]. In the present findings, there was an insignificant effect on the dietary supplementation with REO and GEO on the carcass traits of NZW rabbits. In agreement with the current results, El-Gogary, et al. [51] reported that the dietary supplementation of REO had no positive effect on carcass traits of NZW rabbits. Similarly, feeding diets enriched with peppermint essential oil, basil essential oil, or both did not significantly affect most carcass traits of rabbits [54]. However, the rabbits fed on diets supplemented with oregano extract, rosemary extract, or a combination displayed a significantly higher carcass yield (%) than the control rabbits [3]. Furthermore, nutritional supplementation with thyme essential oil enhanced carcass criteria and reduced perirenal and scapular fat without affecting rabbit internal organs [5]. However, rabbits supplemented with REO and GEO showed significantly higher liver weight percentages and giblets than the control group.

In the current results, the composition of the LD and HL muscles was not significantly affected by the dietary supplementation of REO and GEO to growing rabbits. In agreement with the present findings, diets supplemented with oregano extract, rosemary extract or a combination had no effect on the composition of the hind leg meat of growing rabbits [3]. Similarly, Hemat, et al. [55] found that feeding rabbits on diets containing remnants of mint, fennel, basil, and anise did not alter the chemical composition of the rabbitmeat.

The current findings showed a lowering in cholesterol of both the LD and HL muscles of growing rabbits due to supplementation with rosemary and ginger essential oils. Moreover, there was a significant reduction in the concentration of plasma cholesterol and triglycerides of growing rabbits treated with REO and GEO. The present results were supported by several studies that found that essential oils decreased levels of both cholesterol and triglyceride in rats due to containing limonene, which is the main active component in REO in the present study, as well as citrus EO [31,32,56,57]. Moreover, lemon EO supplementation caused an 18% decrease in triglyceride in rabbits [48]. In addition, ginger EO reduced hepatic lipid accumulation in rats [33]. Moreover, linalool (one of the active components of REO) reduced cholesterol and triglyceride levels [58]. In addition, ginger EO showed lower cholesterol and triglyceride by 21% and 24%, respectively, in male Japanese quail [34] due to the presence of zingiberene, the main constituent in GEO in the present results.

It is noteworthy that high cholesterol is a prevalent problem, as 40% of the world's population has cholesterol levels that are above the recommended limit of 200 g/dL according to the World Health Organization, which could cause severe health problems [48,59,60]. When alternative treatments are used, the risk of side effects of therapeutic drugs for high cholesterol can be minimized [60]. Essential oils contain monoterpenoids and sesquiterpenoids such as 1,8 cineole, citral, farnesol, geraniol, limonene, and linalool, which are emerging as potential lipid-lowering agents with promising cholesterol-lowering effects [60].

In the present study, the observed reduction in cholesterol and triglyceride concentrations of rabbits treated with REO and GEO could be associated with the reduction of hepatic lipid accumulation or the inhibition of the hepatic biosynthesis of cholesterol [60]. Furthermore, the reduction of cholesterol may be due to the regulating effect of terpene derivatives in essential oils on sterol regulatory element-binding protein-1c, which lead to decreased transcription and accelerated degradation of HMG-CoA reductase (statins) as the main cholesterol synthesis pathways [33,60]. Another explanation for reducing cholesterol and triglycerides is stimulating the conversion of cholesterol to bile acids which are excreted from the body through the enterohepatic circulation [61,62]. On the other hand, insignificant effects of REO and GEO supplementation to rabbits on HDL-c, LDL-c plasma levels were found in the present study. Similar to our results, the dietary supplementation of REO did not affect plasma HDL-c or LDL-c in NZW rabbits [51].

In the present study, the supplementation with both REO and GEO at high doses decreased free radical and lipid oxidation in meat by lowering TBARS levels by 10 and 15%, respectively. In accordance with the present results, the dietary supplementation of oregano and rosemary aqueous extracts declined the TBARS concentration of the LD meat compared to the control group, thus resulting in improving the oxidative stability and effectively delaying the lipid oxidation of the LD meat of rabbits [3]. Furthermore, the dietary supplementation with ginger powder decreased the sensitivity of rabbit meat to lipid oxidation, thus offering a promising way to improve rabbit meat quality [35]. Rosemary oil exhibits effective antioxidant activity due to consisting of considerable amounts of limonene, α-pinene, camphor, and (Z)-linalool oxide [63]. Ginger oil has strong antioxidant activities because it contains active compounds including zingiberene, camphene, ar-curcumene, and b-sesquiphellandrene [64].

In muscles and fatty tissues, the oxidation process impacts different constituents, including proteins, carbohydrates, lipids, pigments, vitamins, and DNA. The rate of oxidation rises with time, reducing the shelf-life of meat and meat products [65]. In particular, rabbit meat contains a high content of polyunsaturated fatty acids (the ratio of omega-6/omega-3 = 5.9) that provides a nutritional benefit. However, it also renders the meat more susceptible to lipid oxidation, affecting meat appearance and flavor [66]. In addition, lipid oxidation reduces the healthfulness of meat by causing the development of toxic compounds such as MDA and cholesterol oxidation products, which are harmful to human health [67,68]. The oxidative stability of rabbit meat can be improved by the dietary supplementation with natural antioxidants [2,35].

In addition, the current findings demonstrate that supplementation with GEO at a high dose improved the redox status balance in plasma, by increasing the TAC level by 11.64% and decreasing the MDA level by 7.60% compared to the control. In the same vein, the inclusion of ginger powder and oils in the diet of broiler chickens did not affect blood parameters, but they increased serum TAC levels and lowered MDA more than those of the control group [69].

## 5. Conclusions

In conclusion, the dietary supplementation of rosemary and ginger essential oils, especially at a high dose (0.5%), induced an improvement in the growth performance, feed utilization, and meat quality of the growing NZW rabbits. Body weight gain and feed conversion ratio significantly improved with both rosemary and ginger essential oils supplementation. The levels of cholesterol in muscle and plasma, as well as triglycerides in plasma, were significantly reduced. In addition, muscle fat content tended to decrease in the muscles of rabbits treated with the high level of both essential oils. In addition, rosemary and ginger essential oils attenuated the oxidant and antioxidant balance in the treated animals. This improvement may be reflected positively on rabbit production towards high quality, healthy meat, and sustainable production.

**Author Contributions:** Conceptualization, M.A.E. and A.M.K.; data curation, M.A.E., A.M.K., A.A.E. and S.A.M.; formal analysis, A.M.K. and S.A.M.; investigation M.A.E., A.M.K. and M.M.R.; methodology, M.A.E., A.M.K. and M.M.R.; project administration A.M.K.; resources A.M.K.; software, A.T.M.; visualization, M.A.E., A.M.K., A.E.E. and A.T.M.; validation, M.A.E. and S.A.M.; writing-original draft, M.A.E., A.M.K. and S.A.M.; writing-review and editing, A.E.E., A.A.E., S.A.M. and A.T.M. All authors have read and agreed to the published version of the manuscript.

**Funding:** This work has no funding support.

**Institutional Review Board Statement:** The different protocols applied in this study were approved by the Institutional Animal Care and Use Committees (IACUCs), Pharmaceutical & Fermentation Industries Development Center, City of Scientific Research and Technology Applications, (SRTA-City), Alexandria, Egypt with the approval No: IACUC # 37-6F-1021.

**Informed Consent Statement:** Not applicable.

**Data Availability Statement:** All relevant data are within the paper, and they are available from the corresponding authors.

**Acknowledgments:** Grateful to all the authors involved in the research.

**Conflicts of Interest:** The authors declare no conflict of interest among authors and organizations.

# References

1. Pla, M.; Pascual, M.; Ariño, B. Protein, fat and moisture content of retail cuts of rabbit meat evaluated with the nirs methodology. *World Rabbit Sci.* **2004**, *12*, 149–158. [CrossRef]
2. Zotte, A.D. Perception of rabbit meat quality and major factors influencing the rabbit carcass and meat quality. *Livest. Prod. Sci.* **2002**, *75*, 11–32. [CrossRef]
3. Cardinali, R.; Cullere, M.; Bosco, A.D.; Mugnai, C.; Ruggeri, S.; Mattioli, S.; Castellini, C.; Marinucci, M.T.; Zotte, A.D. Oregano, rosemary and vitamin E dietary supplementation in growing rabbits: Effect on growth performance, carcass traits, bone development and meat chemical composition. *Livest. Sci.* **2015**, *175*, 83–89. [CrossRef]
4. Zotte, A.D.; Szendrő, Z. The role of rabbit meat as functional food. *Meat Sci.* **2011**, *88*, 319–331. [CrossRef]
5. El-Adawy, M.M.; Salem, A.Z.; Khodeir, M.H.; Khusro, A.; Elghandour, M.M.; Hernández, S.R.; Al-Shamandy, O.A. Influence of four tropical medicinal and aromatic plants on growth performance, digestibility, and blood constituents of rabbits. *Agrofor. Syst.* **2020**, *94*, 1279–1289. [CrossRef]
6. Hernández, P.; Zotte, A.D. Influence of diet on rabbit meat quality. In *Nutrition of the Rabbit*; CABI: Worcester, MA, USA, 2010; p. 163.
7. Hernandez, P.; Gondret, F. 5.1 Rabbit meat quality. In *Recent Advances in Rabbit Sciences*; Maertens, L., Coudert, P., Eds.; Institute for Agricultural and Fisheries Research (ILVO): Melle, Belgium, 2006; p. 269.
8. Simopoulos, A. Human requirement for N-3 polyunsaturated fatty acids. *Poult. Sci.* **2000**, *79*, 961–970. [CrossRef]
9. Saini, R.K.; Keum, Y.-S. Omega-3 and omega-6 polyunsaturated fatty acids: Dietary sources, metabolism, and significance—A review. *Life Sci.* **2018**, *203*, 255–267. [CrossRef]
10. Ball, D.M.; Collins, M.; Lacefield, G.; Martin, N.; Mertens, D.; Olson, K.; Putnam, D.; Undersander, D.; Wolf, M. *Understanding Forage Quality*; American Farm Bureau Federation Publication: Washington DC, USA, 2001; Volume 1, p. 21.
11. Madhupriya, V.; Shamsudeen, P.; Manohar, G.R.; Senthilkumar, S.; Soundarapandiyan, V.; Moorthy, M. Phyto Feed Additives in Poultry Nutrition: A Review. *Int. J. Environ. Sci. Technol.* **2018**, *7*, 815–822.
12. Jin, L.-Z.; Dersjant-Li, Y.; Giannenas, I. Application of aromatic plants and their extracts in diets of broiler chickens. In *Feed Additives*; Elsevier: Amsterdam, The Netherlands, 2020; pp. 159–185. [CrossRef]
13. Morshedy, S.A.; Abdelmodather, A.M.; Basyony, M.M.; Zahran, S.A.; Hassan, M.A. Effects of Rocket Seed Oil, Wheat Germ Oil, and Their Mixture on Growth Performance, Feed Utilization, Digestibility, Redox Status, and Meat Fatty Acid Profile of Growing Rabbits. *Agriculture* **2021**, *11*, 662. [CrossRef]
14. Evangelista, A.G.; Corrêa, J.A.F.; Pinto, A.C.S.M.; Luciano, F.B. The impact of essential oils on antibiotic use in animal production regarding antimicrobial resistance–a review. *Crit. Rev. Food Sci. Nutr.* **2021**, 1–17. [CrossRef]
15. Seidavi, A.; Tavakoli, M.; Slozhenkina, M.; Gorlov, I.; Hashem, N.M.; Asroosh, F.; Taha, A.E.; Abd El-Hack, M.E.; Swelum, A.A. The use of some plant-derived products as effective alternatives to antibiotic growth promoters in organic poultry production: A review. *Environ. Sci. Pollut. Res.* **2021**, *28*, 47856–47868. [CrossRef]
16. Al-Suwaiegh, S.B.; Morshedy, S.A.; Mansour, A.T.; Ahmed, M.H.; Zahran, S.M.; Alnemr, T.M.; Sallam, S. Effect of an essential oil blend on dairy cow performance during treatment and post-treatment periods. *Sustainability* **2020**, *12*, 9123. [CrossRef]
17. Ronquillo, M.G.; Hernandez, J.C.A. Antibiotic and synthetic growth promoters in animal diets: Review of impact and analytical methods. *Food Control* **2017**, *72*, 255–267. [CrossRef]
18. Ngangom, B.L.; Tamunjoh, S.S.A.; Boyom, F.F. Antibiotic residues in food animals: Public health concern. *Acta Ecol. Sin.* **2019**, *39*, 411–415.

19. Zeng, Z.; Zhang, S.; Wang, H.; Piao, X. Essential oil and aromatic plants as feed additives in non-ruminant nutrition: A review. *J. Anim. Sci. Biotechnol.* **2015**, *6*, 7–17. [CrossRef] [PubMed]
20. Miguel, M.G. Antioxidant activity of medicinal and aromatic plants. A review. *Flavour Fragr. J.* **2010**, *25*, 291–312. [CrossRef]
21. Oluwafemi, R.; Olawale, I.; Alagbe, J. Recent trends in the utilization of medicinal plants as growth promoters in poultry nutrition-A review. *Res. Agric. Vet. Sci.* **2020**, *4*, 5–11.
22. Abd El-Hack, M.E.; El-Saadony, M.T.; Saad, A.M.; Salem, H.M.; Ashry, N.M.; Ghanima, M.M.A.; Shukry, M.; Swelum, A.A.; Taha, A.E.; El-Tahan, A.M. Essential oils and their nanoemulsions as green alternatives to antibiotics in poultry nutrition: A comprehensive review. *Poult. Sci.* **2021**, *101*, 101584. [CrossRef]
23. Schlieck, T.M.M.; Petrolli, T.G.; Bissacotti, B.F.; Copetti, P.M.; Bottari, N.B.; Morsch, V.M.; da Silva, A.S. Addition of a blend of essential oils (cloves, rosemary and oregano) and vitamin E to replace conventional chemical antioxidants in dog feed: Effects on food quality and health of beagles. *Arch. Anim. Nutr.* **2021**, *75*, 389–403. [CrossRef]
24. Lešnik, S.; Furlan, V.; Bren, U. Rosemary (*Rosmarinus officinalis* L.): Extraction techniques, analytical methods and health-promoting biological effects. *Phytochem. Rev.* **2021**, *20*, 1273–1328. [CrossRef]
25. El-Hack, A.; Mohamed, E.; Alagawany, M.; Shaheen, H.; Samak, D.; Othman, S.I.; Allam, A.A.; Taha, A.E.; Khafaga, A.F.; Arif, M. Ginger and its derivatives as promising alternatives to antibiotics in poultry feed. *Animals* **2020**, *10*, 452. [CrossRef] [PubMed]
26. Mao, Q.-Q.; Xu, X.-Y.; Cao, S.-Y.; Gan, R.-Y.; Corke, H.; Li, H.-B. Bioactive compounds and bioactivities of ginger (*Zingiber officinale* Roscoe). *Foods* **2019**, *8*, 185. [CrossRef] [PubMed]
27. Zhang, M.; Zhao, R.; Wang, D.; Wang, L.; Zhang, Q.; Wei, S.; Lu, F.; Peng, W.; Wu, C. Ginger (*Zingiber officinale* Roscoe) and its bioactive components are potential resources for health beneficial agents. *Phytother. Res.* **2021**, *35*, 711–742. [CrossRef] [PubMed]
28. Mahomoodally, M.; Aumeeruddy, M.; Rengasamy, K.R.; Roshan, S.; Hammad, S.; Pandohee, J.; Hu, X.; Zengin, G. Ginger and its active compounds in cancer therapy: From folk uses to nano-therapeutic applications. *Proc. Semin. Cancer Biol.* **2021**, *69*, 140–149. [CrossRef]
29. Bakr, E.-S.; Ibrahim, I.; Mousa, M.; Shetaewi, M.; Abdel-Samee, A.-S. Rosemary, marjoram and ginger as a feed additives and its influences on growth performance traits of NEZ rabbits under Sainai conditions. *J. Product Dev. (Agri. Res.)* **2016**, *21*, 1–18.
30. Jubril, T.O. Growth Performance and Digestibility in Growing Rabbits Fed Diet Supplemented with Powdered Ginger. *Asian J. Res. Anim. Vet. Sci.* **2019**, *4*, 1–5.
31. Li, D.; Wu, H.; Dou, H. Weight loss effect of sweet orange essential oil microcapsules on obese SD rats induced by high-fat diet. *Biosci. Biotechnol. Biochem.* **2019**, *83*, 923–932. [CrossRef]
32. Lin, L.-Y.; Chuang, C.-H.; Chen, H.-C.; Yang, K.-M. Lime (*Citrus aurantifolia* (Christm.) Swingle) essential oils: Volatile compounds, antioxidant capacity, and hypolipidemic effect. *Foods* **2019**, *8*, 398. [CrossRef]
33. Lai, Y.-S.; Lee, W.-C.; Lin, Y.-E.; Ho, C.-T.; Lu, K.-H.; Lin, S.-H.; Panyod, S.; Chu, Y.-L.; Sheen, L.-Y. Ginger essential oil ameliorates hepatic injury and lipid accumulation in high fat diet-induced nonalcoholic fatty liver disease. *J. Agric. Food Chem.* **2016**, *64*, 2062–2071. [CrossRef]
34. Herve, T.; Raphaël, K.J.; Ferdinand, N.; Vitrice, F.T.L.; Gaye, A.; Outman, M.M.; Marvel, N.M.W. Growth performance, serum biochemical profile, oxidative status, and fertility traits in male Japanese quail fed on ginger (*Zingiber officinale*, Roscoe) essential oil. *Vet. Med. Int.* **2018**, *8*. [CrossRef]
35. Mancini, S.; Secci, G.; Preziuso, G.; Parisi, G.; Paci, G. Ginger (*Zingiber officinale* Roscoe) powder as dietary supplementation in rabbit: Life performances, carcass characteristics and meat quality. *Ital. J. Anim. Sci.* **2018**, *17*, 867–872. [CrossRef]
36. Abouelezz, K.; Abou-Hadied, M.; Yuan, J.; Elokil, A.; Wang, G.; Wang, S.; Wang, J.; Bian, G. Nutritional impacts of dietary oregano and Enviva essential oils on the performance, gut microbiota and blood biochemicals of growing ducks. *Animal* **2019**, *13*, 2216–2222. [CrossRef] [PubMed]
37. Nehme, R.; Andrés, S.; Pereira, R.B.; Jemaa, M.B.; Bouhallab, S.; Ceciliani, F.; López, S.; Rahali, F.Z.; Ksouri, R.; Pereira, D.M. Essential oils in livestock: From health to food quality. *Antioxidants* **2021**, *10*, 330. [CrossRef]
38. NRC. *Nutrient Requirements of Rabbits: 1977*; National Academies Press: Washington, DC, USA, 1977.
39. Villamide, M.; Maertens, L.; de Blas, C. Feed evaluation. In *Nutrition of the Rabbit*, 3rd ed.; Blas, C.D., Wiseman, J., Eds.; CAB International: Wallingford/Oxfordshire, UK, 2020; p. 159.
40. Blasco, A.; Ouhayoun, J. Harmonization of criteria and terminology in rabbit meat research. *World Rabbit Sci.* **1993**, *4*, 93–99. [CrossRef]
41. AOAC. *Association of Official Analytical Chemists. Official Method of Analysis*; AOAC: Gaithersburg, MD, USA, 2006.
42. Dinh, T.; Blanton, J., Jr.; Brooks, J.; Miller, M.; Thompson, L. A simplified method for cholesterol determination in meat and meat products. *J. Food Compost. Anal.* **2008**, *21*, 306–314. [CrossRef]
43. Dal Bosco, A.; Mugnai, C.; Mourvaki, E.; Cardinali, R.; Moscati, L.; Paci, G.; Castellini, C. Effect of genotype and rearing system on the native immunity and oxidative status of growing rabbits. *Ital. J. Anim. Sci.* **2009**, *8*, 781–783. [CrossRef]
44. Koracevic, D.; Koracevic, G.; Djordjevic, V.; Andrejevic, S.; Cosic, V. Method for the measurement of antioxidant activity in human fluids. *J. Clin. Pathol.* **2001**, *54*, 356–361. [CrossRef]
45. Banjare, J.; Salunke, M.; Indapurkar, K.; Ghate, U.; Bhalerao, S. Estimation of serum malondialdehyde as a marker of lipid peroxidation in medical students undergoing examination-induced psychological stress. *J. Sci. Soc.* **2017**, *44*, 137.
46. Duncan, D.B. Multiple range and multiple F-tests. *Biometrics* **1955**, *11*, 1–42. [CrossRef]
47. Zar, J.H. *Biostatistical Analysis*, 2nd ed.; Prentice-Hall, Inc.: Englewood Cliffs, NJ, USA, 1984.

48. Lee, H.; Woo, M.; Kim, M.; Noh, J.S.; Song, Y.O. Antioxidative and cholesterol-lowering effects of lemon essential oil in hypercholesterolemia-induced rabbits. *Prev. Nutr. Food Sci.* **2018**, *23*, 8. [CrossRef]
49. Kiyama, R. Nutritional implications of ginger: Chemistry, biological activities and signaling pathways. *J. Nutr. Biochem.* **2020**, *86*, 108486. [CrossRef] [PubMed]
50. Erdelyi, M.; Matics, Z.; Gerencsér, Z.; Princz, Z.; Szendro, Z.; Mézes, M. Study of the effect of rosemary (*Rosmarinus officinalis*) and garlic (*Allium sativum*) essential oils on the performance of rabbit. In Proceedings of the 9th World Rabbit Congress, Verona, Italy, 10–13 June 2008; pp. 649–654.
51. El-Gogary, M.; El-Said, E.; Mansour, A. Physiological and immunological effects of rosemary essential oil in growing rabbit diets. *J. Agric. Sci.* **2018**, *10*, 485–491. [CrossRef]
52. Jamroz, D.; Wiliczkiewicz, A.; Wertelecki, T.; Orda, J.; Skorupińska, J. Use of active substances of plant origin in chicken diets based on maize and locally grown cereals. *Br. Poult. Sci.* **2005**, *46*, 485–493. [CrossRef] [PubMed]
53. Bento, M.; Ouwehand, A.; Tiihonen, K.; Lahtinen, S.; Nurminen, P.; Saarinen, M.; Schulze, H.; Mygind, T.; Fischer, J. Essential oils and their use in animal feeds for monogastric animals-Effects on feed quality, gut microbiota, growth performance and food safety: A review. *Vet. Med.* **2013**, *58*, 449–458. [CrossRef]
54. Morshedy, S.A.; Zweil, H.S.; Zahran, S.M.; Ahmed, M.H.; El-Mabrok, B.M. Growth performance, carcass traits, immune response and antioxidant status of growing rabbits supplemented with peppermint and basil essential oils. *Egypt. Poult. Sci. J.* **2019**, *39*, 61–79. [CrossRef]
55. Hemat, M.; Mahmoud, A.; Abbas, M.; Sobhy, H. Effects of feeding diets containing of some aromatic and medicinal plants remnants on meat quality, fatty and amino acids fractions of New Zealand white rabbits. *Asian J. Anim. Sci.* **2016**, *10*, 255–261.
56. Costa, C.A.; Cury, T.C.; Cassettari, B.O.; Takahira, R.K.; Flório, J.C.; Costa, M. *Citrus aurantium* L. essential oil exhibits anxiolytic-like activity mediated by 5-HT 1A-receptors and reduces cholesterol after repeated oral treatment. *BMC Complement. Altern. Med.* **2013**, *13*, 42. [CrossRef]
57. Bacanlı, M.; Anlar, H.G.; Aydın, S.; Çal, T.; Arı, N.; Bucurgat, Ü.Ü.; Başaran, A.A.; Başaran, N. D-limonene ameliorates diabetes and its complications in streptozotocin-induced diabetic rats. *Food Chem. Toxicol.* **2017**, *110*, 434–442. [CrossRef]
58. Cho, S.-Y.; Jun, H.-J.; Lee, J.H.; Jia, Y.; Kim, K.H.; Lee, S.-J. Linalool reduces the expression of 3-hydroxy-3-methylglutaryl CoA reductase via sterol regulatory element binding protein-2-and ubiquitin-dependent mechanisms. *FEBS Lett.* **2011**, *585*, 3289–3296. [CrossRef]
59. WHO. *Cholesterol*; World Health Organization: Geneva, Switzerland, 2021.
60. Bahr, T.; Butler, G.; Rock, C.; Welburn, K.; Allred, K.; Rodriguez, D. Cholesterol-lowering activity of natural mono-and sesquiterpenoid compounds in essential oils: A review and investigation of mechanisms using in silico protein–ligand docking. *Phytother. Res.* **2021**, *35*, 4215–4245. [CrossRef]
61. Jun, H.-J.; Lee, J.H.; Jia, Y.; Hoang, M.-H.; Byun, H.; Kim, K.H.; Lee, S.-J. *Melissa officinalis* essential oil reduces plasma triglycerides in human apolipoprotein E2 transgenic mice by inhibiting sterol regulatory element-binding protein-1c–dependent fatty acid synthesis. *J. Nutr.* **2012**, *142*, 432–440. [CrossRef] [PubMed]
62. Hu, G.; Yuan, X.; Zhang, S.; Wang, R.; Yang, M.; Wu, C.; Wu, Z.; Ke, X. Research on choleretic effect of menthol, menthone, pluegone, isomenthone, and limonene in DanShu capsule. *Int. Immunopharmacol.* **2015**, *24*, 191–197. [CrossRef] [PubMed]
63. Jayasena, D.D.; Jo, C. Potential application of essential oils as natural antioxidants in meat and meat products: A review. *Food Rev. Int.* **2014**, *30*, 71–90. [CrossRef]
64. Noori, S.; Zeynali, F.; Almasi, H. Antimicrobial and antioxidant efficiency of nanoemulsion-based edible coating containing ginger (*Zingiber officinale*) essential oil and its effect on safety and quality attributes of chicken breast fillets. *Food Control* **2018**, *84*, 312–320. [CrossRef]
65. Smet, K.; Raes, K.; Huyghebaert, G.; Haak, L.; Arnouts, S.; De Smet, S. Lipid and protein oxidation of broiler meat as influenced by dietary natural antioxidant supplementation. *Poult. Sci.* **2008**, *87*, 1682–1688. [CrossRef] [PubMed]
66. Kone, A.P.N.; Cinq-Mars, D.; Desjardins, Y.; Guay, F.; Gosselin, A.; Saucier, L. Effects of plant extracts and essential oils as feed supplements on quality and microbial traits of rabbit meat. *World Rabbit Sci.* **2016**, *24*, 107–119. [CrossRef]
67. Wood, J.; Richardson, R.; Nute, G.; Fisher, A.; Campo, M.; Kasapidou, E.; Sheard, P.; Enser, M. Effects of fatty acids on meat quality: A review. *Meat Sci.* **2004**, *66*, 21–32. [CrossRef]
68. da Silva Martins, T.; de Lemos, M.V.A.; Mueller, L.F.; Baldi, F.; de Amorim, T.; Ferinho, A.; Muñoz, J.A.; de Souza Fuzikawa, I.H.; de Mouray, G.; Gemelli, J.L. Fat deposition, fatty acid composition, and its relationship with meat quality and human health. In *Meat Science and Nutrition*; Arshad, M.S., Ed.; BoD-Books on Demand: Norderstedt, Germany, 2018; pp. 17–37.
69. Habibi, R.; Sadeghi, G.; Karimi, A. Effect of different concentrations of ginger root powder and its essential oil on growth performance, serum metabolites and antioxidant status in broiler chicks under heat stress. *Br. Poult. Sci.* **2014**, *55*, 228–237. [CrossRef] [PubMed]

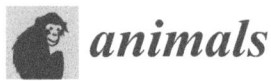

Article

# Dietary Supplementation with Goji Berries (*Lycium barbarum*) Modulates the Microbiota of Digestive Tract and Caecal Metabolites in Rabbits

Paola Cremonesi [1,†], Giulio Curone [2], Filippo Biscarini [1,†], Elisa Cotozzolo [3], Laura Menchetti [4,\*], Federica Riva [2], Maria Laura Marongiu [5], Bianca Castiglioni [1], Olimpia Barbato [6], Albana Munga [7], Marta Castrica [8], Daniele Vigo [2], Majlind Sulce [7], Alda Quattrone [6], Stella Agradi [2,\*] and Gabriele Brecchia [2]

1. Institute of Agricultural Biology and Biotechnology (IBBA), National Research Council (CNR), U.O.S. di Lodi, Via Einstein, 26900 Lodi, Italy; cremonesi@ibba.cnr.it (P.C.); biscarini@ibba.cnr.it (F.B.); castiglioni@ibba.cnr.it (B.C.)
2. Department of Veterinary Medicine, University of Milano, Via dell'Università 6, 26900 Lodi, Italy; giulio.curone@unimi.it (G.C.); federica.riva@unimi.it (F.R.); daniele.vigo@unimi.it (D.V.); gabriele.brecchia@unimi.it (G.B.)
3. Department of Agricultural, Food and Environmental Sciences, University of Perugia, Borgo XX Giugno 74, 06121 Perugia, Italy; elisa.cotozzolo@studenti.unipg.it
4. Department of Agricultural and Food Sciences, University of Bologna, Viale G. Fanin 44, 40137 Bologna, Italy
5. Department of Veterinary Medicine, University of Sassari, Via Vienna, 2, 07100 Sassari, Italy; marongiu@uniss.it
6. Department of Veterinary Medicine, University of Perugia, Via San Costanzo 4, 06126 Perugia, Italy; olimpia.barbato@unipg.it (O.B.); alda.quattrone@hotmail.it (A.Q.)
7. Faculty of Veterinary Medicine, Agricultural University of Tirana, Kodër-Kamëz, 1029 Tirana, Albania; amunga@ubt.edu.al (A.M.); msulce@ubt.edu.al (M.S.)
8. Department of Health, Animal Science and Food Safety "Carlo Cantoni", University of Milan, Via dell'Università 6, 26900 Lodi, Italy; marta.castrica@unimi.it
\* Correspondence: laura.menchetti7@gmail.com (L.M.); stella.agradi@unimi.it (S.A.)
† These authors contributed equally to this work.

**Simple Summary:** The microbial community that inhabits specific areas of the body, developing a symbiotic relationship with the host, is termed the microbiota. The intestinal microbiota plays a pivotal role in different physiological processes and is influenced by many factors, including nutrition. Goji berries are a popular nutraceutical product that have been proposed as a dietary supplement in some livestock species, including rabbits, but their effects on the composition of the microbiota have never been investigated. This study evaluated the effects of Goji berry supplementation on the microbiota of different digestive tracts (stomach, duodenum, jejunum, ileum, caecum and colon) of the rabbit, using a modern method of analysis. Our results suggest that Goji berries could modulate the microbiota of the rabbit's digestive tract increasing the growth of beneficial bacteria, such as Ruminococcaceae, Lachnospiraceae, Lactobacillaceae, and particularly, the genus *Lactobacillus*. These findings suggest that Goji berries could be used to produce innovative feeds for rabbits, although further studies are necessary to evaluate their impact on productive performance, gut immune system maturation, as well as resistance to gastrointestinal disorders.

**Abstract:** Goji berries show health benefits, although the possible mechanisms of action, including compositional changes in the gut microbiome, are still not fully understood. The aim of this study was to evaluate the effect of Goji berry supplementation on microbiota composition and metabolites in the digestive tracts of rabbits. Twenty-eight New Zealand White rabbits were fed with a commercial feed (control group, C; $n = 14$) or the same diet supplemented with 3% of Goji berries (Goji group, G; $n = 14$), from weaning (35 days old) until slaughter (90 days old). At slaughter, samples from the content of the gastrointestinal tracts were collected and analyzed by Next Generation 16S rRNA Gene Sequencing to evaluate the microbial composition. Ammonia and lactic acid were also quantified in caecum. Results showed differences in microbiota composition between the groups for two phyla (Cyanobacteria and Euryarchaeota), two classes (Methanobacteria and Bacilli), five orders, fourteen

---

Citation: Cremonesi, P.; Curone, G.; Biscarini, F.; Cotozzolo, E.; Menchetti, L.; Riva, F.; Marongiu, M.L.; Castiglioni, B.; Barbato, O.; Munga, A.; et al. Dietary Supplementation with Goji Berries (*Lycium barbarum*) Modulates the Microbiota of Digestive Tract and Caecal Metabolites in Rabbits. *Animals* **2022**, *12*, 121. https://doi.org/10.3390/ani12010121

Academic Editors: Iveta Plachá, Monika Pogány Simonová and Andrea Lauková

Received: 29 November 2021
Accepted: 3 January 2022
Published: 5 January 2022

**Publisher's Note:** MDPI stays neutral with regard to jurisdictional claims in published maps and institutional affiliations.

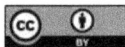

Copyright: © 2022 by the authors. Licensee MDPI, Basel, Switzerland. This article is an open access article distributed under the terms and conditions of the Creative Commons Attribution (CC BY) license (https:// creativecommons.org/licenses/by/ 4.0/).

families, and forty-five genera. Ruminococcaceae ($p < 0.05$) and Lachnospiraceae ($p < 0.01$) were more abundant in G than in C group. Lactobacillaceae also showed differences between the two groups, with *Lactobacillus* as the predominant genus ($p = 0.002$). Finally, Goji berry supplementation stimulated lactic acid fermentation ($p < 0.05$). Thus, Goji berry supplementation could modulate gastrointestinal microbiota composition and caecal fermentation.

**Keywords:** Goji fruit; intestinal bacterial community; caecum; lactic acid; ammonium; rabbit

## 1. Introduction

Goji berries, the fruits of the *Lycium barbarum* plant, are often used in traditional Chinese medicine for their nutritional and therapeutic properties, and are also widespread as supplementation in Western diets [1,2]. Their health benefits are associated with biologically active compounds, including polysaccharides, carotenoids, polyphenols, amino acids, ascorbic acid, and unsaturated fatty acids [3], although their mechanisms of action are still not fully understood. Recent evidence has shown that the fruit could modulate the gut microbiota and thus have a role in the prevention and treatment of several gastrointestinal diseases in mice [4,5], rats [6] and humans [7]. Recently, Goji berries have also been proposed as a dietary supplement for some livestock species, with the dual aim of improving productive performance and product quality [8–10]. In rabbits, Goji berry supplementation seems to improve reproductive [11] and productive performances, [12] energy metabolism [13], and meat quality [14,15] in a dose-dependent manner, but its effects on gut microbiota have not yet been investigated.

The microbiota represents a complex ecosystem of microorganisms which inhabits specific niches of the body and plays important roles in physiological processes developing symbiotic relationships with the host [16]. The intestinal microbiota is involved in the digestion and absorption of nutrients, maturation and stimulation of the immune system, as well as protection against pathogenic infections [17]. The bacterial microbiota composition along the gastrointestinal tract of adult rabbits fed with a commercial diet has recently been characterized [18]. This study showed interesting differences among the various sections of the digestive system in bacterial richness and diversity [18]. Within the same species, however, bacterial community composition of the gastrointestinal tract can be influenced by several factors, including nutrition [13]. Goji supplementation could therefore induce favorable changes in the intestinal microbiota of the rabbit with beneficial effects on health and productive performance, as seen in other animal species and humans [4–10].

The rabbit is a very interesting species because it can be a pet, livestock or animal model. Both in pet and farmed rabbits, the digestive system is a common site of diseases that are often associated with changes in intestinal microbiota [19,20]. In particular, the peri-weaning period is the most critical physiological phase as the diet transition induces changes in the gut microbiota increasing sensitivity to gastrointestinal pathogens [21]. Antibiotics are commonly used to control intestinal infections; however, according to recommendations of the European Union, this practice should be reduced [22,23]. An innovative strategy to limit the incidence of gastrointestinal disorders could be the use of specific feeds for pet and farmed rabbits integrated with nutraceutical products such, as *Lycium barbarum* fruit, to favor the growth of a beneficial gut microbiota. Understanding the effects of Goji berry supplementation on the intestinal microbiota can therefore have important implications for the health of rabbits. The rabbit could be also considered as an animal model for diet-induced changes in gut microbiota, as it has already been used for studies exploring the effect of nutrition on productive [24–26], reproductive [27,28], and immunological traits [29,30].

The aim of this study was to investigate the effect of Goji berry supplementation on the microbiota composition of the different tracts of the digestive system (stomach, duodenum, jejunum, ileum, caecum, and colon) in the rabbit. For this purpose, the microbiota of all the sections of the digestive apparatus was analyzed using Next Generation 16S rRNA Gene Sequencing. In addition, metabolites from bacterial fermentation in the caecum (lactic acid and ammonia) were also quantified.

## 2. Materials and Methods

### 2.1. Animals and Samples Collection

The experimental trial was conducted in the facilities of the Faculty of Veterinary Medicine of the Agricultural University of Tirana, Tirana, Albania.

The rabbits were maintained under the supervision of a responsible veterinarian and in accordance with the Directive 2010/63/EU regarding the protection of animals kept for farming purposes. The lowest number of rabbits necessary to obtain reliable results was used for the trial.

According to dietary treatment, 28 New Zealand White male rabbits were randomly assigned into two groups from weaning (35 days of age) until slaughter (90 days of age): control group (n = 14 animals, C), fed with a commercial pellet, and Goji group (n = 14 animals, G), fed with the same feed of the C group supplemented with 3% of Goji berries (Gianluca Bazzica, Foligno, Italy) before pelleting (Table 1). At weaning the average body weight was 875 ± 115 g and 893 ± 135 in C and G groups, respectively. Feeds from the same batches were previously used in other experiments [11,13–15].

Table 1. Feed formulation and chemical composition (as fed) of control group and Goji group diet.

| Ingredients | Unit | Diet | |
|---|---|---|---|
| | | Control | Goji |
| Wheat bran | % | 30.0 | 29.0 |
| Dehydrated alfalfa meal | % | 42.0 | 41.0 |
| Barley | % | 9.5 | 9.0 |
| Sunflower meal | % | 4.5 | 4.2 |
| Rice bran | % | 4.0 | 3.9 |
| Soybean meal | % | 4.0 | 3.9 |
| Calcium carbonate | % | 2.2 | 2.2 |
| Cane molasses | % | 2.0 | 2.0 |
| Dicalcium phosphate | % | 0.7 | 0.7 |
| Vitamin-mineral premix [1] | % | 0.4 | 0.4 |
| Soybean oil | % | 0.4 | 0.4 |
| Salt | % | 0.3 | 0.3 |
| Goji berries | % | - | 3.0 |
| Chemical composition | | | |
| Crude Protein | % | 15.74 | 15.66 |
| Ether extract | % | 2.25 | 2.47 |
| Ash | % | 9.28 | 9.25 |
| Starch | % | 16.86 | 16.99 |
| NDF | % | 38.05 | 37.49 |
| ADF | % | 19.54 | 19.01 |
| ADL | % | 4.01 | 3.98 |
| Digestible Energy [2] | MJ/Kg | 10.3 | 10.3 |

[1] Per kg diet: vitamin A 11,000 IU; vitamin D3 2000 IU; vitamin B1 2.5 mg; vitamin B2 4 mg; vitamin B6 1.25 mg; vitamin B12 0.01 mg; alpha-tocopherol acetate 50 mg; biotine 0.06 mg; vitamin K 2.5 mg; niacin 15 mg; folic acid 0.30 mg; D-pantothenic acid 10 mg; choline 600 mg; Mn 60 mg; Fe 50 mg; Zn 15 mg; I 0.5 mg; Co 0.5 mg. [2] NDF: Neutral Detergent Fiber; ADF: Acid Detergent Fiber; ADL: Acid Detergent Lignin. Estimated by Maertens et al. [31].

Rabbits were bred in single cages and maintained at a temperature range between 18 and 21 °C, relative humidity of 60%, and with a photoperiod of 16 h of light. Throughout the entire trial, water and feed were provided ad libitum.

At the slaughterhouse, the gastrointestinal tract was immediately removed from each rabbit. The content of the different digestive tract sections from each animal (stomach, duodenum, jejunum, ileum, caecum, and colon) were collected separately in 15 mL sterile tubes and then stored at −80 °C until examination. Each sample was analyzed individually. The average body weights (±standard error) at weaning were 875 ± 55 g and 893 ± 75, while at slaughter, they were 2310 ± 82 g and 2357 ± 82 g in C and G groups, respectively.

*2.2. Microbiota Evaluation—Genomic Sequencing*

2.2.1. DNA Extraction

Using the commercial QIAamp PowerFecal Pro DNA Kit (Qiagen, Hilden, Germany), the bacterial DNA was extracted from each sample of intestinal contents following the manufacturer's protocol. DNA quality and quantity were checked using a NanoDrop ND-1000 spectrophotometer (NanoDrop Technologies, Wilmington, DE, USA, and the obtained DNA was stoked at −20 °C until use.

2.2.2. 16S Ribosomal RNA (rRNA) Gene Sequencing

Bacterial DNA was amplified using primers described in the literature [32] which target the V3-V4 hypervariable regions of the 16S rRNA gene. All the PCR amplifications were performed in 25 µL volumes per sample. A total of 12.5 µL of KAPA HIFI Master Mix 2× (Kapa Biosystems, Inc., Wilmington, MA, USA) and 0.2 µL of each primer (100 µM) were added to 2 µL of genomic DNA (5 ng/µL). Blank controls (no DNA template added to the reaction) were also performed. A first amplification step was performed in an Applied Biosystem 2700 thermal cycler (ThermoFisher Scientific, Waltham, MA, USA). The samples were denatured at 95 °C for 3 min, followed by 25 cycles with a denaturing step at 98 °C for 30 s, annealing at 56 °C for 1 min, and extension at 72 °C for 1 min, with a final extension at 72 °C for 7 min. The amplicons were then cleaned with Agencourt AMPure XP (Beckman, Coulter Brea, CA, USA), and libraries were prepared following the 16S Metagenomic Sequencing Library Preparation Protocol (Illumina, San Diego, CA, USA). The libraries obtained were quantified using Real Time PCR with KAPA Library Quantification Kits (Kapa Biosystems, Inc., Wilmington, MA, USA), pooled in equimolar proportion, and then sequenced in one MiSeq (Illumina, San Diego, CA, USA) run with 2 × 250-base paired-end reads.

2.2.3. Sequence Analysis

The reads obtained by the 16S rRNA sequencing were analyzed as previously described [18]. One rabbit from the Goji group and two samples, both from G diet (caecum intestinal tract), were removed because they had a total number of counts <100.

2.2.4. Alpha and Beta Diversity Indices

To assess the microbial diversity of the different rabbit gastrointestinal tracts the alpha (within-) and beta (across-) diversities were used. These indices were estimated starting from the OTU table, after filtering with more than 50 total counts, distributed in at least five samples. Besides the number of observed OTUs directly, within-sample microbial richness, diversity, and evenness were estimated using Chao1 and ACE (abundance-based coverage estimator) for richness, Shannon, Simpson, and Fisher's alpha for diversity [33,34], and Simpson E and Pielou's J (Shannon's evenness) for evenness [35]. The Bray–Curtis dissimilarity [36] was used to quantify the across-sample microbiota diversity. Prior to the calculation of these metrics, the OTU counts were normalized for uneven sequencing depth by cumulative sum scaling (CSS) [37]. Details of these analyses can be found in Biscarini et al. [38].

2.2.5. Software

The QIIME 1.9 pipeline [39] was utilized both to analyze the reads obtained from 16S rRNA gene sequencing and to estimate most diversity indices. Own Python (https://github.com/filippob/Rare-OTUs-ACE.git, accessed on 15 November 2021) and R (https://github.com/filippob/sampleBasedRarefaction, accessed on 15 November 2021) scripts were used to estimate the ACE index and sample-based rarefaction. The figures were generated with the ggplot2 R package [40]. The R environment for statistical computing [41] was used to perform the additional data handling and statistical analysis.

### 2.3. Lactic Acid and Ammonia Quantification

For the analysis of bacterial metabolites (lactic acid and ammonia), 1 g of caecal content was diluted in 1 mL of 1 M perchloric acid and 8 mL of distilled water. After homogenization, tubes were centrifuged for 10 min at 5000 rpm, and the supernatant was transferred to 2 mL Eppendorf tube and frozen at $-20\,°C$ until metabolite quantification. The spectrophotometric method for biological fluids was used for lactic acid determination in accordance with Pryce et al. [42]. Ammonia concentration was detected in line with Patton et al. [43]. Spectrophotometer was set at 565 nm and 660 nm respectively (Shimadzu Corporation UV-2550, Kyoto, Japan). All chemicals were purchased from Sigma Chemical Co (St. Louis, MO, USA).

### 2.4. Statistical Analysis

Differences in alpha diversity indexes between treatments at various taxonomic levels along the rabbit's gastrointestinal tract were tested with a linear model that took into account the hierarchical structure of within-subject nested data (consecutive sections of the gastrointestinal tract belonging to individual rabbits). The model had the following form:

$$y_{ijkt} = \mu + rabbit_j + treatment_k + anatomic\ region_{t(j)} + e_{ijkt} \quad (1)$$

where $y_{ijkt}$ is the alpha diversity index value for record i from rabbit j with treatment k and anatomic region t, $\mu$ is the intercept, $rabbit_j$ is the systematic effect of the individual rabbits, $treatment_k$ is the treatment effect (Goji vs. control), anatomic $region_{tk(j)}$ is the effect of the anatomic region of the gastrointestinal tract nested within $rabbit_j$, and $e_{ijkt}$ is the residual.

$$Var(y) = Sigma + I\sigma_e^2$$

where Sigma is a block diagonal matrix, with 1 s on the diagonal and the covariances $\sigma_{ij}$ between records within rabbits in the off-diagonal block elements, I is the identity matrix, and $\sigma_e^2$ is the residual variance.

A simplified version of Model (1) was used to evaluate differences between Goji and control samples; in particular, where the anatomic region effect was dropped and data from all gastrointestinal sections were analyzed jointly to evaluate the effect of Goji supplementation on the overall rabbit gut microbiota.

For Bray–Curtis dissimilarities (beta diversity), differences along the digestive tract were tested non-parametrically using the permutational analysis of variance approach (999 permutations; [33]).

## 3. Results

### 3.1. Sequencing Results

The microbiota structure of the gastrointestinal tract of C and G groups was characterized by a total of 6,122,359 and 7,156,769 high quality reads (after filtering), respectively, with a mean of 75,584 ± 38,864 reads for C and 90,592 ± 33,296 reads for G group. The evaluation of the sample-based and sequence-based rarefaction curves suggested that the depth of coverage was sufficient to describe the biological diversity within the samples (Figure S1).

### 3.2. Taxonomic Composition of Gut Microbiota along the Rabbit Gastrointestinal Tract of C and G Groups

Phylum relative abundances distribution along the gastrointestinal tract of C and G groups are summarized in Figure 1. Significative differences were found in microbiota composition between the experimental groups for two phyla, two classes, five orders, fourteen families, and forty-five genera (Table S1). Firmicutes represented the main phylum in all sections of the digestive tract, especially in the most distal portions of caecum and colon (77–79% of total bacteria) for both groups, and Bacteroidetes the second (14–16% of total bacteria). The caecum and colon of rabbits treated with Goji berries showed differences regarding the abundance of Bacteroidetes (16%) compared to the control group (14%) although these were not statistically significant. As regards other phyla, Actinobacteria was present in the upper part of the gastrointestinal tract. In the jejunum, its relative abundance was higher in C than G group (7.5% for C vs. 5.5% for G group), while in the ileum the percentages were opposite (4.8% for C vs. 5.2% for G group); as with the Bacteroidetes, the differences regarding Actinobacteria were not significant. On the other hand, at the phylum level, Cyanobacteria and Euryarchaeota, the latter belonging to kingdom Archaea, were statistically different ($p = 0.034$ and $p = 0.004$, respectively) between the experimental groups, with higher relative abundances in the upper part of the gastrointestinal tract in G group.

Moreover, Clostridia represented the major class in all anatomic regions, while Ruminococcaceae and Lachnospiraceae were the most abundant families in the Goji group (Figure 2).

Figure 3 shows the comparison of the relative abundances of significant OTUs between treatments and along the rabbit's gastrointestinal tract. As shown in Table S1 and Figure 3, there were significant differences between the groups; Bacillales were predominant ($p = 0.0032$) in the G group, and *Bacillus* was the major genus in the stomach ($p = 0.0036$). Ruminococcaceae UCG-005, Lachnospiraceae NK4B4 group, and Christensenellaceae R-7 group were genera detected in all the digestive tracts with statistically significant different results between the groups. As reported in Table S1, the Lactobacillaceae family was significantly different ($p = 0.0018$) between the groups with *Lactobacillus* as the predominant genus in G group compared to C group.

*3.3. F/B Ratio*

The Firmicutes: Bacteroidetes (F:B) ratio followed a clear pattern along the rabbit's digestive tract starting at around 10 in the stomach, increasing clearly in the duodenum and jejunum, and finally decreasing again in the caecum and colon. The F:B ratio appeared to be significantly lower in the G group (Figure 4), in the duodenum ($p = 0.0176$) and jejunum ($p = 0.000049$). This was confirmed by bootstrapping (1000 replicates resampled with replacement from the original data, Figure 5), which provided further statistical support of the significance of F:B differences between G and C groups in the duodenum, jejunum and, slightly less so, in the ileum.

*3.4. Alpha Diversity Index—Treatment by Region*

Table 2 reports the values for the alpha diversity indexes estimated in the rabbits' gastrointestinal tract, in the two groups. Alpha diversity indexes were significantly different between treatments in the last portion of the digestive tract (Figure S2): six indexes were significantly different in the jejunum (ACE, Fisher's alpha, observed n. of OTUs, Shannon and Simpson diversity), two in the ileum (Equitability and Simpson E), three in the caecum (Chao1, ACE, Fisher's alpha), and two in the colon (Equitability and Simpson E).

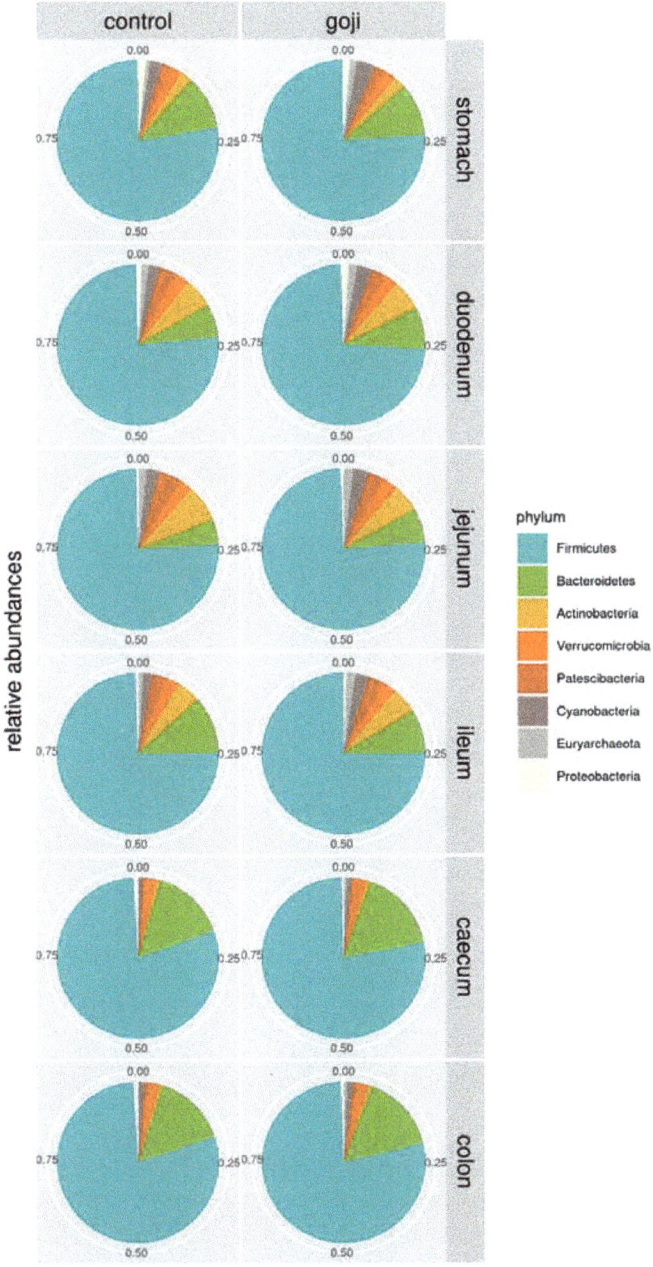

**Figure 1.** Pie-chart of phylum relative abundances in control and Goji-treated rabbits along the gastrointestinal tract. For the analyses, 14 and 13 samples were used for the control and Goji groups, respectively.

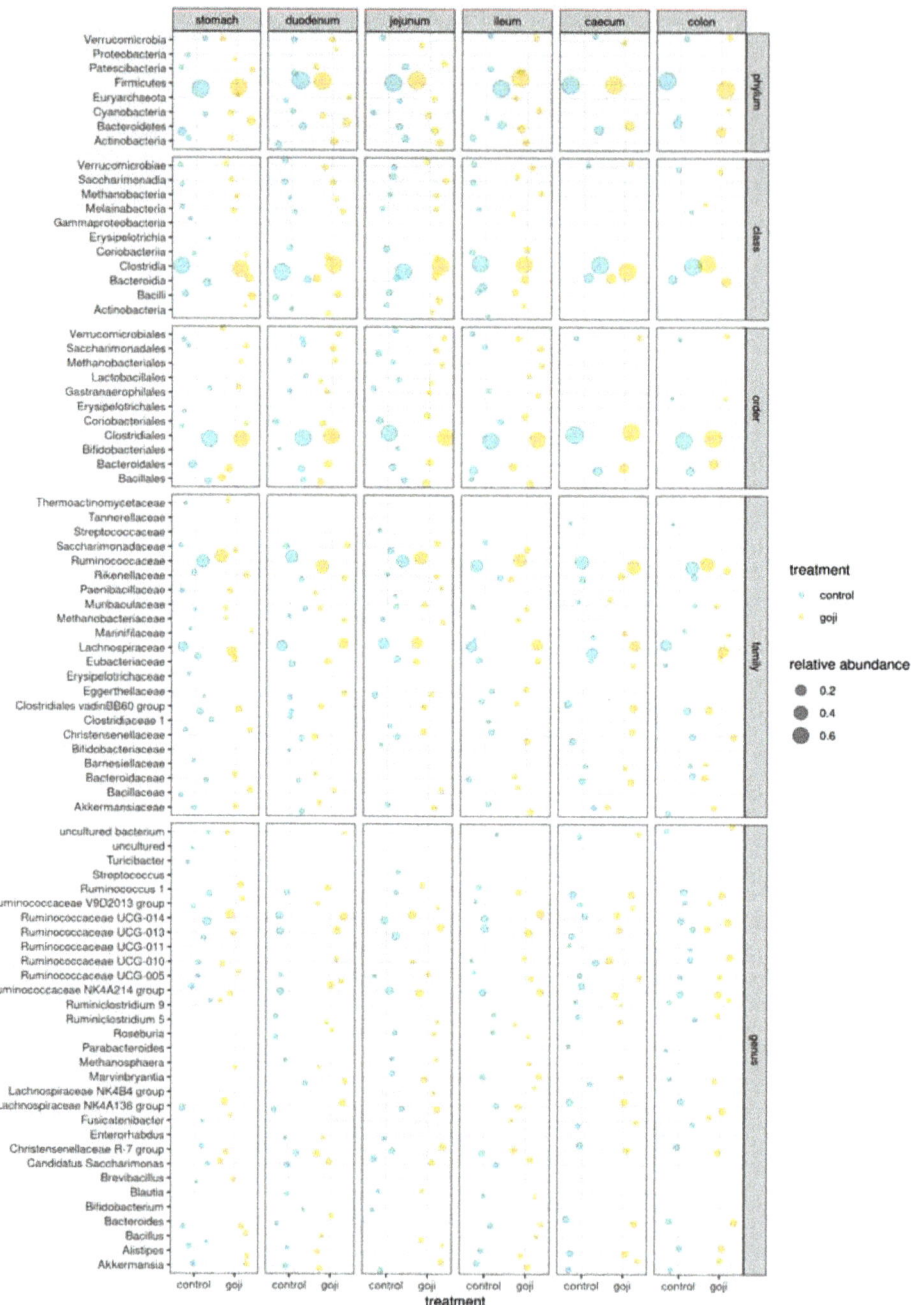

**Figure 2.** Bubble chart of relative abundances of all taxa (≥1%) in the microbiota of the digestive tract of rabbits, grouped by taxonomic level. Control (blue = 14 rabbits) and Goji (yellow = 13 rabbits) experimental groups. The size of the bubble is proportional to the relative abundance, with 0.2, 0.4 and 0.6 hallmarks, as shown in the legend.

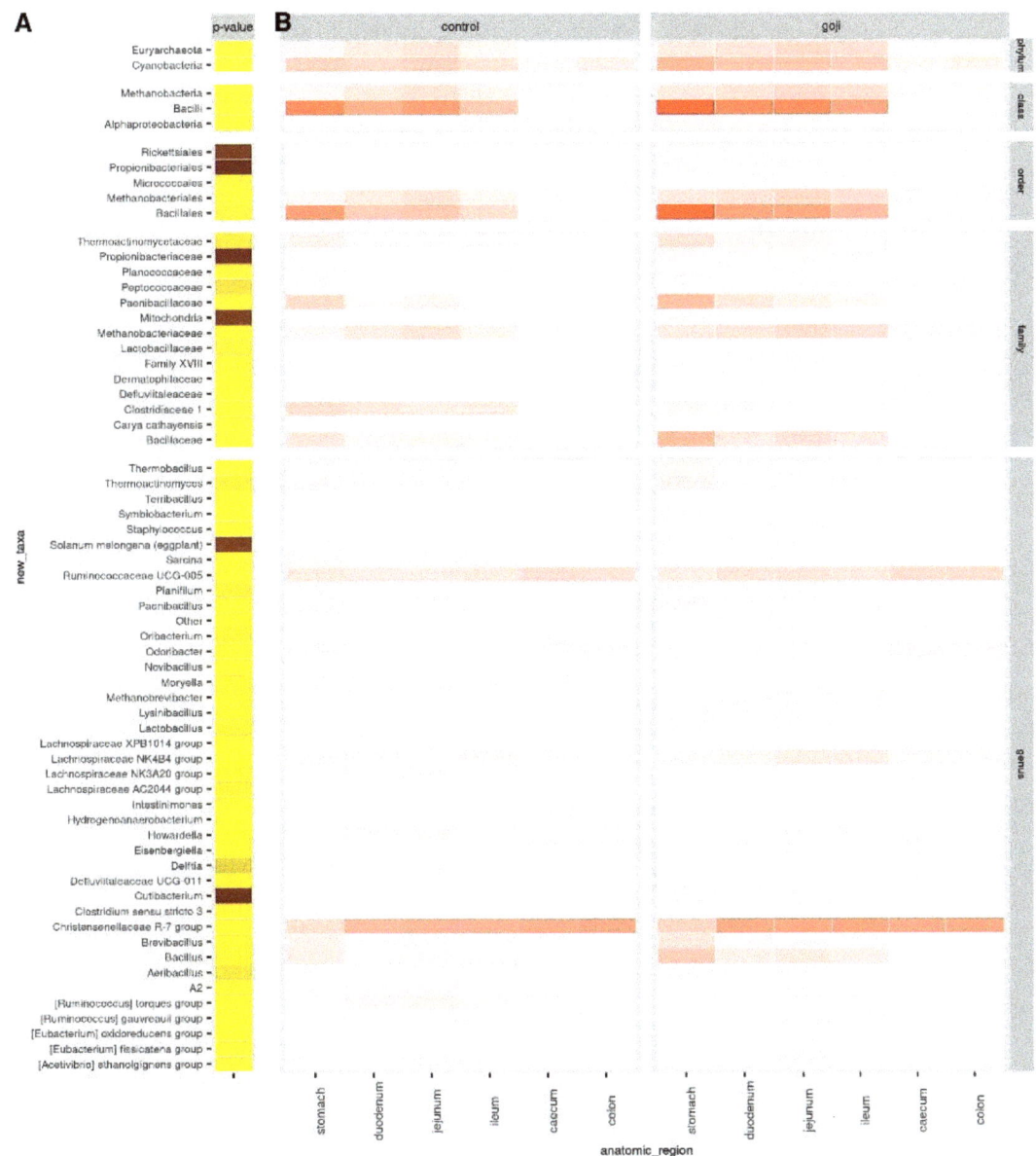

**Figure 3.** Significantly different OTUs. OTU significantly different between treatments from analysis of variance based on normalized counts: $p$-values (**A**) and counts per group and anatomic region of the rabbit digestive tract (**B**). $p$-value < 0.05 was used as cut-off. Darker colours indicate lower $p$-values (**A**) or higher counts (**B**). $p$-values are in the range $10^{-15}$–0.049, from dark brown to light yellow. For the analyses, 14 and 13 samples were used for the control and Goji groups, respectively.

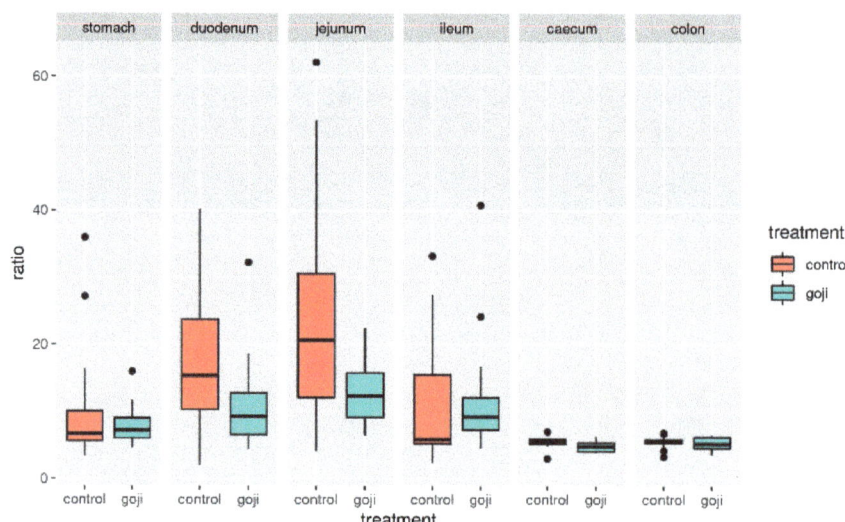

**Figure 4.** Distribution of the F:B ratio (Firmicutes to Bacteroidetes) in control and Goji-treated groups along the gastrointestinal tract. For the analyses, 14 and 13 samples were used for the control and Goji groups, respectively.

**Table 2.** Alpha diversity indices along the digestive tract of rabbits in the two experimental groups (14 controls and 13 Goji-treated; two more samples, both from caecum intestinal G diet were removed because they had a total number of read counts < 100). * indicates significant difference ($p < 0.05$) between control and Goji groups.

| Group | Anatomic Portion | N | Chao1 | Ace | Fisher Alpha | Observed OTUS | Shannon | Simpson | Equitability | Simpson E |
|---|---|---|---|---|---|---|---|---|---|---|
| Control | Stomach | 14 | 378.115 | 380.038 | 163.32 | 335.786 | 7.779 | 0.993 | 0.973 | 0.747 |
| Goji | Stomach | 13 | 320.39 | 318.117 | 135.593 | 300.923 | 7.926 | 0.995 | 0.976 | 0.766 |
| Control | Duodenum | 14 | 279.333 | 274.565 | 120.298 | 268.143 | 7.806 | 0.995 | 0.976 | 0.764 |
| Goji | Duodenum | 13 | 329.489 | 325.595 | 142.572 | 312.462 | 7.999 | 0.995 | 0.975 | 0.750 |
| Control | Jejunum | 14 | 205.000 * | 205.000 * | 85.734 * | 205.000 * | 7.427 * | 0.993 * | 0.979 | 0.787 |
| Goji | Jejunum | 13 | 306.591 * | 305.284 * | 130.950 * | 287.000 * | 7.878 * | 0.995 * | 0.975 | 0.750 |
| Control | Ileum | 14 | 341.365 | 345.910 | 152.660 | 327.286 | 8.034 | 0.995 | 0.975 * | 0.749 * |
| Goji | Ileum | 13 | 410.027 | 396.468 | 169.947 | 355.000 | 8.149 | 0.996 | 0.968 * | 0.700 * |
| Control | Caecum | 14 | 683.149 * | 640.207 * | 274.313 * | 534.714 | 8.734 | 0.997 | 0.965 | 0.674 |
| Goji | Caecum | 11 | 553.633 * | 555.73 * | 235.517 * | 494.909 | 8.642 | 0.997 | 0.966 | 0.687 |
| Control | Colon | 14 | 621.580 | 616.796 | 271.393 | 529.929 | 8.731 | 0.997 | 0.966 * | 0.682 * |
| Goji | Colon | 13 | 656.245 | 638.687 | 265.692 | 543.385 | 8.744 | 0.997 | 0.964 * | 0.666 * |

### 3.5. Beta Diversity Index (Clustering Treatment X Anatomic Portion)

Figure 6a shows the clustering of samples (C and G groups) from Bray–Curtis dissimilarities (first three dimensions from non-metric multidimensional scaling). The distance between groups were significantly different ($p < 0.01$) from permutational multivariate analysis of variance (PERMANOVA, 999 permutations). This difference appeared to vary along the gastrointestinal tract, with jejunum, caecum, and colon showing the clearest differences, while the two groups mostly overlapped in the stomach, duodenum, and ileum (Figure 6b: first two NMDS dimensions only).

### 3.6. Caecal Lactic Acid and Ammonia Quantification

Regarding lactic acid quantification, G group showed a higher concentration than C group, suggesting higher bacterial activity (3.91 ± 1.59 and 1.01 ± 1.22 mmol/kg in C and G groups, respectively; $p = 0.033$). No significant differences in ammonia concentration were detected between the two groups (5.81 ± 2.22 and 5.89 ± 1.81 mmol/kg in C and G groups, respectively; $p = 0.305$).

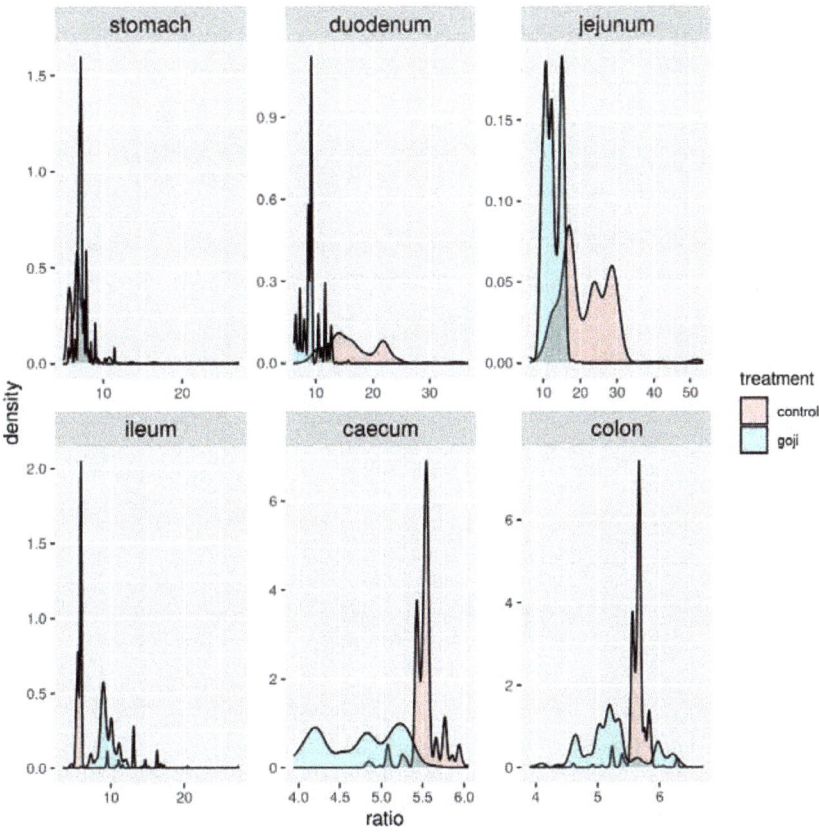

**Figure 5.** Distribution of the F:B ratio (x-axis) along the digestive tract in Goji-treated (blue) and control (red) rabbits from 1000 bootstrapping replicates of the data. For the analyses, 14 and 13 samples were used for the control and Goji groups, respectively.

(a)

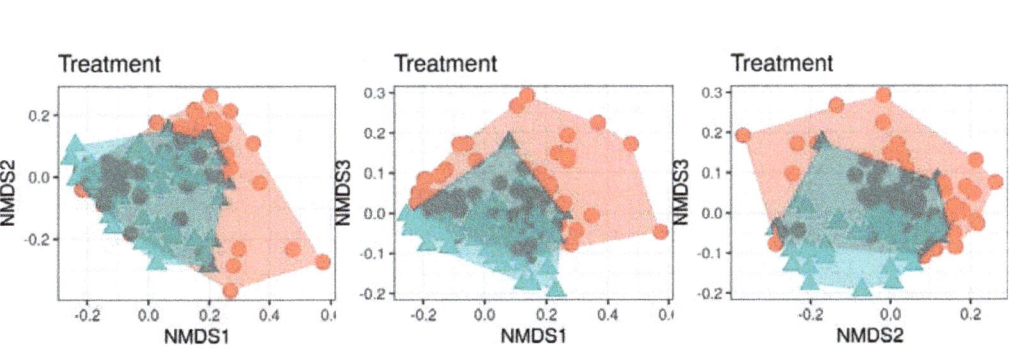

**Figure 6.** *Cont.*

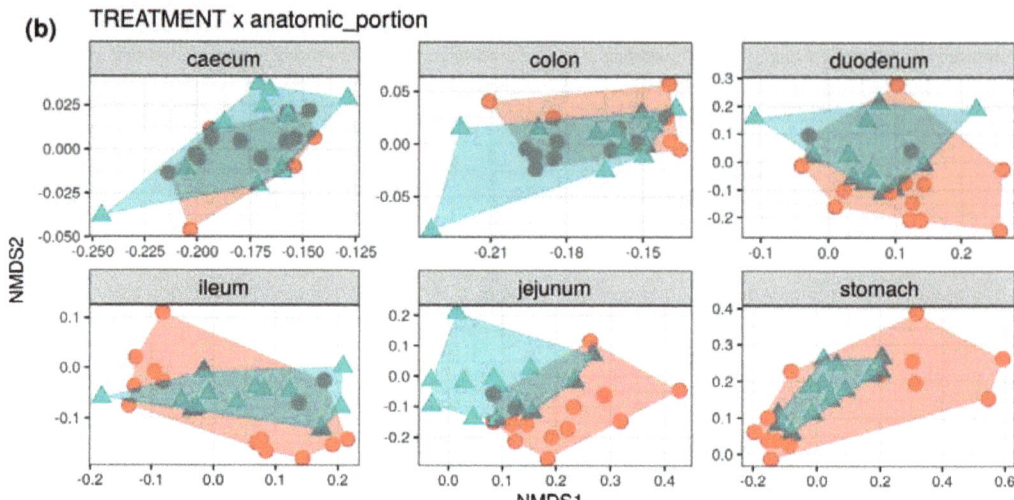

**Figure 6.** (**a**): Non-metric multidimensional scaling plot of Bray-Curtis dissimilarities estimated from the OTU table. The plots show the first three NMDS dimensions (from left to right: dimensions one and two, one and three, two and three). Control samples in red circles, Goji-treated samples in blue triangles. (**b**): First two dimensions from the non-metric dimensional scaling of Bray-Curtis dissimilarities between control and Goji-treated samples along the digestive tract of rabbits. For the analyses, 14 and 11–13 samples were used for the control and Goji groups, respectively.

## 4. Discussion

Diet is one of the main factors affecting the composition of the microbiota in the digestive tract due to the relation between nutrients and microbial populations [44]. The bacterial populations inhabiting the different gastrointestinal compartments of the rabbit have been previously described [18]. For the first time, this study investigated the effect of Goji berry supplementation on microbiota composition in the different tracts of the digestive system and on caecal bacterial fermentations of adult rabbits.

The results of the present study showed a prevalence of Firmicutes in all the anatomic tracts in both experimental groups. This phylum is classified as the most efficient cellulose degrader [45] and it plays a fundamental role in rabbit digestion. Similar results were reported by both Cotozzolo et al. [18] and Arazzuria et al. [46]. This result was also supported by other studies investigating not only the caecal microbiota of rabbits [47,48] but also the gastrointestinal content and feces of both wild and domestic rabbits [49]. This is a common condition not only in hindgut fermenters, such as rabbits, but also in ruminants and monogastric animals [50].

Bacteroidetes was the second most abundant phylum, especially in the large intestine (caecum and colon tracts), and was slightly predominant in the G group. This phylum, not significantly different between the two groups and along the digestive tracts, is known for its role in the stimulation of gut-associated lymphoid tissue [46,48]. The abundance of Bacteroidetes is in accordance with what was already observed by Cotozzolo et al. [18] on the rabbit gastrointestinal microbiota and by Crowley et al. [49] on both domestic and wild rabbits. A further analysis of our samples with a shotgun metagenomic or metatranscriptomic approach, combined with immunological assays, could provide more information about the role of this relevant phylum in gut immunity.

Regarding other phyla, Verrucomicrobia were found in all sections, while Actinobacteria and Proteobacteria were found in the stomach and small intestine. Although with low levels in the core microbiome, the Euryarchaeota phylum, belonging to the kingdom

Archea, was statistically different between the two groups, with higher levels in the G group in all the digestive tracts. All species of this phylum were taxonomically assigned to the methanogenic genus *Methanobrevibacter* [51]. Though this phylum is not very common in the intestinal microflora of some species, such as horses and pigs [18], it is often found in the human gut with the role of increasing polysaccharide digestion by consuming the end products of bacterial fermentation [52].

Clostridia, anaerobic Gram-positive bacteria present in the intestinal microbiota of human, mouse, chicken, and pig, represented the major class in all anatomic regions, in accordance with Velasco-Galilea and co-workers [51]; they are prevalent, cellulose-degrading symbiotic microorganisms, helping the rabbit for plant material digestion [51].

The families of Ruminococcaceae and Lachnospiraceae were present in all anatomic parts, and both were higher in the G group. Ruminococcaceae are usually prevalent in healthy rabbits [53], while Lachnospiraceae is known to be associated with a decrease of mortality [54]. These two families appear to have an important role in fiber digestion, in particular of peptose and cellulose [55], and are significant producers of short-chain fatty acids [56]. Moreover, as previously reported [4], in mice a diet with Goji supplementation promotes butyrate-producing bacteria, including Lachnospiraceae and Ruminococcaceae families, preventing colitis; their high levels in the digestive apparatus also allow protective and beneficial effects towards different diseases, such as diabetes and heart disease [57].

Lactobacillaceae was another family that showed significant differences between the two groups, although present in small quantities. Within this family, *Lactobacillus* was the predominant genus. Lactobacilli are rare in the rabbit intestine, occupying less than 1% of the total intestinal bacteria [58], and their function in gut health is not fully understood. A recent study has shown that the total intestinal bacteria from rabbits tends to induce a higher inflammatory level than the total intestinal bacteria from chickens or pigs [59], probably because of the low abundance of Lactobacilli in the rabbit's intestine. Thus, the higher *Lactobacillus* abundance in rabbits supplemented with Goji could play a protective role against inflammatory diseases. Components of commensal bacteria can alleviate intestinal inflammation by regulating the expression of both pro-inflammatory and anti-inflammatory factors. Kawashima et al. [60] reported that bacterial double-stranded RNA, abundant in *Lactobacillus bacteria*, showed a regulatory function by triggering anti-inflammatory factor IFN-β production and inhibiting pro-inflammatory factors production.

The F:B ratio was at around 10 in the stomach, then increased in the duodenum and jejunum, and subsequently progressively decreased from the ileum to the caecum and colon. The F:B ratio appeared to be lower in the G group, significantly so in the duodenum and jejunum, less so in the ileum, caecum and colon, as also shown by the bootstrapping analysis. Studies in human microbiota and in animal models, have reported that the F:B ratio was directly related to body weight modifications and in particular to obesity [61]. In obese people, the population of Firmicutes shows an elevated proportion with a reduced Bacteroidetes population; this unbalance causes an altered F:B ratio [62]. Additionally, a strong correlation between the F:B ratio and milk fat yield has been observed in dairy cattle [63]. In previous studies, feed supplementation in livestock has been reported to alter the F:B ratio in the gut microbiota (e.g., grape pomace supplementation in cattle [38]). Further studies could investigate the link between Goji intake, F:B ratio and lipid metabolism in rabbits.

The alpha diversity results revealed higher microbial richness and diversity in bacterial composition independently from the treatments in the large intestine. That was an expected result because, as already demonstrated in other livestock species, the microbial densities (and also diversity) along the gastrointestinal tract is maximal in the fermenting compartments [64]. Indeed, Cotozzolo et al. found alpha diversity of the cecum and colon to be significantly higher than for the other compartments of the rabbit gastrointestinal tract [18]. As previously reported [18], this variability, typical of colon and caecum tracts, is due essentially to their physiological functions, such as fermentation of cellulose with production of volatile fatty acids (VFA) and their absorption for energy production. Goji berry supplementation caused higher microbial richness, especially in the jejunum, ileum, and colon tracts, where six indexes were significantly different in the jejunum (ACE, Fisher's alpha, observed n. of OTUs, Shannon and Simpson diversity), two in the ileum (Equitability and Simpson E), three in the caecum (Chao1, ACE, Fisher's alpha), and two in the colon (Equitability and Simpson E). In particular, the principal families involved in the microbial richness were Ruminococcaceae and Lachnospiraceae, as well as *Lactobacillus* spp. These conditions could guarantee greater resilience toward dysbiosis in the gut microbiota, which is necessary to maintain homeostasis and, in turn, the healthy status of the gastrointestinal system [65]. The beta diversity was greatly influenced by Goji treatment, especially in caecum and colon tracts, which play fundamental roles in the digestion of fermenter animals, such as rabbits. Conversely, less influence of this treatment was found in the stomach, duodenum, and ileum tracts.

The differences in microbiota composition are due to the environmental conditions, such as pH modifications, along the gastrointestinal tract. In adult rabbits, the principal substrates for caecal microorganisms are polysaccharides and protein. Caecal microorganisms ferment available nutrients, converting them to metabolites (e.g., short-chain VFA, ammonia, $H_2$, $CH_4$, $CO_2$) and compounds that are incorporated into microbial cells [66]. Our results for caecal bacterial fermentations indicate that Goji berry supplementation did not influence proteolytic activity and ammonia production. On the other hand, Goji supplementation stimulated lactic acid fermentation, indicating changes in the intestinal microbiota in favor of specific bacterial populations. The caecum represents the main site of fermentative activity in the rabbit due to the presence of an abundant microbial flora [1]. Rabbits produce large amounts of VFA and lactate by fermentation of dietary carbohydrates, such as xylan and pectin, in the hindgut [67–69]. Lactobacilli are strong producers of lactic acid and, for this reason, can compete against pathogenic bacteria [70]. Regarding Goji berry supplementation, several authors [71,72] have confirmed the beneficial effects of this integration on the physiology and health of the gut acting on the intestinal microbiota composition of human and mice. Castrica et al. [15] reported that the incorporation of 3% w/w of Goji berries in the rabbit diet was able to increase the Lactobacilli population in rabbit meat.

This is a preliminary study on the effect of Goji berry supplementation on gastrointestinal microbiota of the rabbit and, although its practical implications are currently limited, it may represent a starting point for future exploratory research. Further experimental trials could be addressed to evaluate whether caecal fermentative activities (VFA production) could be affected by changes in microbial community composition. Moreover, evaluation of digestive efficiency by performing an in vivo digestibility trial could integrate the study of the microbiota composition of the rabbit. Finally, it could be interesting to evaluate the impact of microbiota modification on the maturation and activity of the immune system, as well as on resistance to infectious diseases, animal welfare and the productive performance of the rabbit.

## 5. Conclusions

The present study demonstrated that Goji berry supplementation can modulate gastrointestinal microbiota composition and caecal fermentations of the rabbit. In particular, *Lycium barbarum* fruit increased the growth of the phylum Bacteroidetes as well as of Ruminococcaceae, Lachnospiraceae, and *Lactobacillus* in the caecum and colon, and as a consequence, lactic acid production. The mechanism of absorption and integration of the bioactive molecules contained in the fruit, and their influence on the microbiota population, should be investigated to appropriately use Goji berries' probiotic properties. The use of this natural compound needs to be further studied for its implications for both commercial performance and animal resistance to infection, as its supplementation could reduce the incidence of health problems in livestock and consequent antibiotic treatments.

**Supplementary Materials:** The following are available online at https://www.mdpi.com/article/10.3390/ani12010121/s1: Figure S1: Evaluation of the sample-based and sequence-based bacterial rarefaction curves to check the depth of coverage; Figure S2: *p*-values for the difference in alpha diversity indices between control and Goji-treated rabbits, along the gastrointestinal tract; Table S1: Significantly different OTUs between Goji-treated and control rabbits in the gut microbiota ($p < 0.05$).

**Author Contributions:** Conceptualization, L.M., D.V. and G.B.; data curation, P.C., F.B., L.M., B.C., O.B. and M.C.; formal analysis, G.C., F.B., L.M., M.L.M., O.B. and G.B.; funding acquisition, P.C., M.L.M., B.C., D.V. and G.B.; investigation, G.C., E.C., A.M., M.C., M.S. and S.A.; methodology, P.C., E.C., B.C., A.M. and S.A.; project administration, L.M., M.L.M., A.M. and G.B.; resources, F.R., M.L.M., D.V. and G.B.; software, F.B. and L.M.; supervision, P.C., O.B., D.V., M.S. and G.B.; validation, P.C., F.B., F.R. and G.B.; visualization, F.B., B.C. and A.Q.; writing—original draft, P.C., G.C., F.B., E.C., L.M., F.R., M.L.M., A.Q., S.A. and G.B.; writing—review and editing, G.C., L.M., A.M., A.Q., S.A. and G.B. All authors have read and agreed to the published version of the manuscript.

**Funding:** This research was supported by FAR 2019 of the University of Sassari.

**Institutional Review Board Statement:** The Albanian Ministry of Agriculture and Rural Development, National Authority of Veterinary and Plants protection authorized the protocol of the experimental trial (prot. 824/2021).

**Data Availability Statement:** The data presented in this study are available in the article and Supplementary materials. Further information is available upon request from the corresponding author.

**Acknowledgments:** The authors gratefully acknowledge the collaboration and support of Giovanni Migni.

**Conflicts of Interest:** The authors declare no conflict of interest.

# References

1. Yao, X.; Peng, Y.; Xu, L.J.; Li, L.; Wu, Q.L.; Xiao, P.G. Phytochemical and biological studies of lycium medicinal plants. *Chem. Biodivers.* **2011**, *8*, 976–1010. [CrossRef]
2. Sun, W.; Shahrajabian, M.H.; Cheng, Q. Therapeutic Roles of Goji Berry and Ginseng in Traditional Chinese. *J. Nutr. Food Secur.* **2019**, *4*, 293–305. [CrossRef]
3. Magiera, S.; Zaręba, M. Chromatographic determination of phenolic acids and flavonoids in *Lycium barbarum* L. and evaluation of antioxidant activity. *Food Anal. Methods* **2015**, *8*, 2665–2674. [CrossRef]
4. Kang, Y.; Yang, G.; Zhang, S.; Ross, C.F.; Zhu, M.J. Goji Berry Modulates Gut Microbiota and Alleviates Colitis in IL-10-Deficient Mice. *Mol. Nutr. Food Res.* **2018**, *62*, e1800535. [CrossRef]
5. Ding, Y.; Yan, Y.; Chen, D.; Ran, L.; Mi, J.; Lu, L.; Jing, B.; Li, X.; Zeng, X.; Cao, Y. Modulating effects of polysaccharides from the fruits of: *Lycium barbarum* on the immune response and gut microbiota in cyclophosphamide-treated mice. *Food Funct.* **2019**, *10*, 3671–3683. [CrossRef] [PubMed]
6. Hsieh, S.Y.; Lian, Y.Z.; Lin, I.H.; Yang, Y.C.; Tinkov, A.A.; Skalny, A.V.; Chao, J.C.J. Combined Lycium babarum polysaccharides and C-phycocyanin increase gastric Bifidobacterium relative abundance and protect against gastric ulcer caused by aspirin in rats. *Nutr. Metab.* **2021**, *18*, 4. [CrossRef] [PubMed]
7. Pap, N.; Fidelis, M.; Azevedo, L.; do Carmo, M.A.V.; Wang, D.; Mocan, A.; Pereira, E.P.R.; Xavier-Santos, D.; Sant'Ana, A.S.; Yang, B.; et al. Berry polyphenols and human health: Evidence of antioxidant, anti-inflammatory, microbiota modulation, and cell-protecting effects. *Curr. Opin. Food Sci.* **2021**, *42*, 167–186. [CrossRef]
8. Chen, J.; Long, L.; Jiang, Q.; Kang, B.; Li, Y.; Yin, J. Effects of dietary supplementation of *Lycium barbarum* polysaccharides on growth performance, immune status, antioxidant capacity and selected microbial populations of weaned piglets. *J. Anim. Physiol. Anim. Nutr.* **2020**, *104*, 1106–1115. [CrossRef] [PubMed]
9. Bai, X.; Yan, X.; Xie, L.; Hu, X.; Lin, X.; Wu, C.; Zhou, N.; Wang, A.; See, M.T. Effects of pre-slaughter stressor and feeding preventative Chinese medicinal herbs on glycolysis and oxidative stability in pigs. *Anim. Sci. J.* **2016**, *87*, 1028–1033. [CrossRef] [PubMed]
10. Chen, H.; Guo, B.; Yang, M.; Luo, J.; Hu, Y.; Qu, M. Response of Growth Performance, Blood Biochemistry Indices, and Rumen Bacterial Diversity in Lambs to Diets Containing Supplemental Probiotics and Chinese Medicine Polysaccharides. *Front. Vet. Sci.* **2021**, *8*, 656. [CrossRef]
11. Andoni, E.; Curone, G.; Agradi, S.; Barbato, O.; Menchetti, L.; Vigo, D.; Zelli, R.; Cotozzolo, E.; Ceccarini, M.R.; Faustini, M.; et al. Effect of Goji Berry (*Lycium barbarum*) Supplementation on Reproductive Performance of Rabbit Does. *Animals* **2021**, *11*, 1672. [CrossRef]
12. Menchetti, L.; Vecchione, L.; Filipescu, I.; Petrescu, V.F.; Fioretti, B.; Beccari, T.; Ceccarini, M.R.; Codini, M.; Quattrone, A.; Trabalza-Marinucci, M.; et al. Effects of Goji berries supplementation on the productive performance of rabbit. *Livest. Sci.* **2019**, *220*, 123–128. [CrossRef]

13. Menchetti, L.; Curone, G.; Andoni, E.; Barbato, O.; Troisi, A.; Fioretti, B.; Polisca, A.; Codini, M.; Canali, C.; Vigo, D.; et al. Impact of goji berries (*Lycium barbarum*) supplementation on the energy homeostasis of rabbit does: Uni- and multivariate approach. *Animals* **2020**, *10*, 2000. [CrossRef]
14. Menchetti, L.; Brecchia, G.; Branciari, R.; Barbato, O.; Fioretti, B.; Codini, M.; Bellezza, E.; Trabalza-Marinucci, M.; Miraglia, D. The effect of Goji berries (*Lycium barbarum*) dietary supplementation on rabbit meat quality. *Meat Sci.* **2020**, *161*, 108018. [CrossRef]
15. Castrica, M.; Menchetti, L.; Balzaretti, C.M.; Branciari, R.; Ranucci, D.; Cotozzolo, E.; Vigo, D.; Curone, G.; Brecchia, G.; Miraglia, D. Impact of dietary supplementation with goji berries (*Lycium barbarum*) on microbiological quality, physico-chemical, and sensory characteristics of rabbit meat. *Foods* **2020**, *9*, 1480. [CrossRef] [PubMed]
16. Flint, H.J.; Scott, K.P.; Louis, P.; Duncan, S.H. The role of the gut microbiota in nutrition and health. *Nat. Rev. Gastroenterol. Hepatol.* **2012**, *9*, 577–589. [CrossRef] [PubMed]
17. Bagóné Vantus, V.; Kovacs, M.; Zsolnai, A. The rabbit caecal microbiota: Development, composition and its role in the prevention of digestive diseases—A review on recent literature in the light of molecular genetic methods. *Acta Agrar. Kvar.* **2014**, *18*, 55–65.
18. Cotozzolo, E.; Cremonesi, P.; Curone, G.; Menchetti, L.; Riva, F.; Biscarini, F.; Marongiu, M.L.; Castrica, M.; Castiglioni, B.; Miraglia, D.; et al. Characterization of bacterial microbiota composition along the gastrointestinal tract in rabbits. *Animals* **2020**, *11*, 31. [CrossRef]
19. Reusch, B. Rabbit gastroenterology. *Vet. Clin. N. Am. Exot. Anim. Pract.* **2005**, *8*, 351–375. [CrossRef]
20. Chen, H.-J.; Yang, W.-Y.; Wang, C.-Y. The Review on the Function of Intestinal Flora and the Regulatory Effects of Probiotics on the Intestinal Health of Rabbits. Advances in Biological Sciences Research (ABSR). In *Advances in Biological Sciences Research, Proceedings of the 2017 2nd International Conference on Biological Sciences and Technology (BST 2017), Zhuhai, China, 17–19 November 2017*; Atlantis Press: Amsterdam, The Netherlands, 2017; Volume 6, ISBN 978-94-6252-472-9.
21. Chevance, A.; Moulin, G. *Suivi des Ventes de Médicaments Vétérinaires Contenant des Antibiotiques en France en 2007*; AFSSA-ANMV: Javené, France, 2009; pp. 1–44.
22. Nogacka, A.M.; Salazar, N.; Arboleya, S.; Suárez, M.; Fernández, N.; Solís, G.; de los Reyes-Gavilán, C.G.; Gueimonde, M. Early microbiota, antibiotics and health. *Cell. Mol. Life Sci.* **2018**, *75*, 83–91. [CrossRef]
23. Marshall, B.M.; Ochieng, D.J.; Levy, S.B. Commensals: Underappreciated reservoir of antibiotic resistance. *Microbe* **2009**, *4*, 231–238. [CrossRef]
24. Rommers, J.M.; Boiti, C.; Brecchia, G.; Meijerhof, R.; Noordhuizen, J.P.T.M.; Decuypere, E.; Kemp, B. Metabolic adaptation and hormonal regulation in young rabbit does during long-term caloric restriction and subsequent compensatory growth. *Anim. Sci.* **2004**, *79*, 255–264. [CrossRef]
25. Menchetti, L.; Brecchia, G.; Canali, C.; Cardinali, R.; Polisca, A.; Zerani, M.; Boiti, C. Food restriction during pregnancy in rabbits: Effects on hormones and metabolites involved in energy homeostasis and metabolic programming. *Res. Vet. Sci.* **2015**, *98*, 7–12. [CrossRef] [PubMed]
26. Martínez-Paredes, E.; Ródenas, L.; Martínez-Vallespín, B.; Cervera, C.; Blas, E.; Brecchia, G.; Boiti, C.; Pascual, J.J. Effects of feeding programme on the performance and energy balance of nulliparous rabbit does. *Animal* **2012**, *6*, 1086–1095. [CrossRef]
27. Brecchia, G.; Menchetti, L.; Cardinali, R.; Castellini, C.; Polisca, A.; Zerani, M.; Maranesi, M.; Boiti, C. Effects of a bacterial lipopolysaccharide on the reproductive functions of rabbit does. *Anim. Reprod. Sci.* **2014**, *147*, 128–134. [CrossRef] [PubMed]
28. Boiti, C.; Canali, C.; Brecchia, G.; Zanon, F.; Facchin, E. Effects of induced endometritis on the life-span of corpora lutea in pseudopregnant rabbits and incidence of spontaneous uterine infections related to fertility of breeding does. *Theriogenology* **1999**, *52*, 1123–1132. [CrossRef]
29. Boiti, C.; Guelfi, G.; Zerani, M.; Zampini, D.; Brecchia, G.; Gobbetti, A. Expression patterns of cytokines, p53 and nitric oxide synthase isoenzymes in corpora lutea of pseudopregnant rabbits during spontaneous luteolysis. *Reproduction* **2004**, *127*, 229–238. [CrossRef] [PubMed]
30. Collodel, G.; Moretti, E.; Brecchia, G.; Kuželová, L.; Arruda, J.; Mourvaki, E.; Castellini, C. Cytokines release and oxidative status in semen samples from rabbits treated with bacterial lipopolysaccharide. *Theriogenology* **2015**, *83*, 1233–1240. [CrossRef] [PubMed]
31. Maertens, L.; Moermans, R.; De Groote, G. The influence of the dietary energy content on the performances of post-partum breeding does. *J. Appl. Rabbit Res.* **1988**, *11*, 60–67.
32. Caporaso, J.G.; Lauber, C.L.; Walters, W.A.; Berg-Lyons, D.; Lozupone, C.A.; Turnbaugh, P.J.; Fierer, N.; Knight, R. Global patterns of 16S rRNA diversity at a depth of millions of sequences per sample. *Proc. Natl. Acad. Sci. USA* **2011**, *108*, 4516–4522. [CrossRef]
33. Fisher, R.A.; Corbet, A.S.; Williams, C.B. The Relation Between the Number of Species and the Number of Individuals in a Random Sample of an Animal Population. *J. Anim. Ecol.* **1943**, *12*, 42. [CrossRef]
34. Chao, A. Nonparametric estimation of the number of classes in a population. *Scand. J. Stat.* **1984**, *11*, 265–270.
35. Smith, B.; Wilson, J.B. A Consumer's Guide to Evenness Indices. *Oikos* **1996**, *76*, 70. [CrossRef]
36. Bray, J.R.; Curtis, J.T. An Ordination of the Upland Forest Communities of Southern Wisconsin. *Ecol. Monogr.* **1957**, *27*, 325–349. [CrossRef]
37. Paulson, J.N.; Colin Stine, O.; Bravo, H.C.; Pop, M. Differential abundance analysis for microbial marker-gene surveys. *Nat. Methods* **2013**, *10*, 1200–1202. [CrossRef]
38. Biscarini, F.; Palazzo, F.; Castellani, F.; Masetti, G.; Grotta, L.; Cichelli, A.; Martino, G. Rumen microbiome in dairy calves fed copper and grape-pomace dietary supplementations: Composition and predicted functional profile. *PLoS ONE* **2018**, *13*, e0205670. [CrossRef] [PubMed]

39. Caporaso, J.G.; Kuczynski, J.; Stombaugh, J.; Bittinger, K.; Bushman, F.D.; Costello, E.K.; Fierer, N.; Pẽa, A.G.; Goodrich, J.K.; Gordon, J.I.; et al. QIIME allows analysis of high-throughput community sequencing data. *Nat. Methods* **2010**, *7*, 335–336. [CrossRef] [PubMed]
40. Wickham, H. *Ggplot2 Elegant Graphics for Data Analysis*; Springer: Berlin/Heidelberg, Germany, 2016; ISBN 3319242776.
41. Team, R.D.C. *A Language and Environment for Statistical Computing*; R Foundation for Statistical Computing: Vienna, Austria, 2018; Volume 2.
42. Pryce, J.D. A modification of the Barker-Summerson method for the determination of lactic acid. *Analyst* **1969**, *94*, 1151–1152. [CrossRef] [PubMed]
43. Patton, C.J.; Crouch, S.R. Spectrophotometric and Kinetics Investigation of the Berthelot Reaction for the Determination of Ammonia. *Anal. Chem.* **1977**, *49*, 469. [CrossRef]
44. Xu, Z.; Knight, R. Dietary effects on human gut microbiome diversity. *Br. J. Nutr.* **2015**, *113*, S1–S5. [CrossRef]
45. Abecia, L.; Rodríguez-Romero, N.; Yañez-Ruiz, D.R.; Fondevila, M. Biodiversity and fermentative activity of caecal microbial communities in wild and farm rabbits from Spain. *Anaerobe* **2012**, *18*, 344–349. [CrossRef]
46. Arrazuria, R.; Pérez, V.; Molina, E.; Juste, R.A.; Khafipour, E.; Elguezabal, N. Diet induced changes in the microbiota and cell composition of rabbit gut associated lymphoid tissue (GALT). *Sci. Rep.* **2018**, *8*, 14103. [CrossRef]
47. Abecia, L.; Fondevila, M.; Balcells, J.; Edwards, J.E.; Newbold, C.J.; McEwan, N.R. Molecular profiling of bacterial species in the rabbit caecum. *FEMS Microbiol. Lett.* **2005**, *244*, 111–115. [CrossRef]
48. Monteils, V.; Cauquil, L.; Combes, S.; Godon, J.J.; Gidenne, T. Potential core species and satellite species in the bacterial community within the rabbit caecum. *FEMS Microbiol. Ecol.* **2008**, *66*, 620–629. [CrossRef]
49. Crowley, E.J.; King, J.M.; Wilkinson, T.; Worgan, H.J.; Huson, K.M.; Rose, M.T.; McEwan, N.R. Comparison of the microbial population in rabbits and guinea pigs by next generation sequencing. *PLoS ONE* **2017**, *12*, e0165779. [CrossRef] [PubMed]
50. Zhao, W.; Wang, Y.; Liu, S.; Huang, J.; Zhai, Z.; He, C.; Ding, J.; Wang, J.; Wang, H.; Fan, W.; et al. The dynamic distribution of porcine microbiota across different ages and gastrointestinal tract segments. *PLoS ONE* **2015**, *10*, e0117441. [CrossRef] [PubMed]
51. Velasco-Galilea, M.; Piles, M.; Viñas, M.; Rafel, O.; González-Rodríguez, O.; Guivernau, M.; Sánchez, J.P. Rabbit microbiota changes throughout the intestinal tract. *Front. Microbiol.* **2018**, *9*, 2144. [CrossRef] [PubMed]
52. Horz, H.P.; Conrads, G. The discussion goes on: What is the role of Euryarchaeota in humans? *Archaea* **2010**, *2010*, 967271. [CrossRef]
53. Morrow, A.L.; Lagomarcino, A.J.; Schibler, K.R.; Taft, D.H.; Yu, Z.; Wang, B.; Altaye, M.; Wagner, M.; Gevers, D.; Ward, D.V.; et al. Early microbial and metabolomic signatures predict later onset of necrotizing enterocolitis in preterm infants. *Microbiome* **2013**, *1*, 13. [CrossRef]
54. Combes, S.; Gidenne, T.; Cauquil, L.; Bouchez, O.; Fortun-Lamothe, L. Coprophagous behavior of rabbit pups affects implantation of cecal microbiota and health status. *J. Anim. Sci.* **2014**, *92*, 652–665. [CrossRef]
55. Gosalbes, M.J.; Durbán, A.; Pignatelli, M.; Abellan, J.J.; Jiménez-Hernández, N.; Pérez-Cobas, A.E.; Latorre, A.; Moya, A. Metatranscriptomic approach to analyze the functional human gut microbiota. *PLoS ONE* **2011**, *6*, e17447. [CrossRef]
56. Zhu, Y.; Wang, C.; Li, F. Impact of dietary fiber/starch ratio in shaping caecal microbiota in rabbits. *Can. J. Microbiol.* **2015**, *61*, 771–784. [CrossRef]
57. Zeng, X.; Gao, X.; Peng, Y.; Wu, Q.; Zhu, J.; Tan, C.; Xia, G.; You, C.; Xu, R.; Pan, S.; et al. Higher Risk of Stroke Is Correlated with Increased Opportunistic Pathogen Load and Reduced Levels of Butyrate-Producing Bacteria in the Gut. *Front. Cell. Infect. Microbiol.* **2019**, *9*, 4. [CrossRef]
58. Yu, B.; Tsen, H.Y. *Lactobacillus* cells in the rabbit digestive tract and the factors affecting their distribution. *J. Appl. Bacteriol.* **1993**, *75*, 269–275. [CrossRef]
59. Cui, H.X.; Xu, X.R. Comparing the effect of intestinal bacteria from rabbit, pig, and chicken on inflammatory response in cultured rabbit crypt and villus. *Can. J. Microbiol.* **2019**, *65*, 59–67. [CrossRef] [PubMed]
60. Kawashima, T.; Kosaka, A.; Yan, H.; Guo, Z.; Uchiyama, R.; Fukui, R.; Kaneko, D.; Kumagai, Y.; You, D.J.; Carreras, J.; et al. Double-Stranded RNA of Intestinal Commensal but Not Pathogenic Bacteria Triggers Production of Protective Interferon-β. *Immunity* **2013**, *38*, 1187–1197. [CrossRef] [PubMed]
61. Turnbaugh, P.J.; Ley, R.E.; Mahowald, M.A.; Magrini, V.; Mardis, E.R.; Gordon, J.I. An obesity-associated gut microbiome with increased capacity for energy harvest. *Nature* **2006**, *444*, 1027–1031. [CrossRef] [PubMed]
62. Mariat, D.; Firmesse, O.; Levenez, F.; Guimarães, V.D.; Sokol, H.; Doré, J.; Corthier, G.; Furet, J.P. The Firmicutes/Bacteroidetes ratio of the human microbiota changes with age. *BMC Microbiol.* **2009**, *9*, 123. [CrossRef]
63. Jami, E.; White, B.A.; Mizrahi, I. Potential role of the bovine rumen microbiome in modulating milk composition and feed efficiency. *PLoS ONE* **2014**, *9*, e85423. [CrossRef]
64. Yeoman, C.J.; White, B.A. Gastrointestinal tract microbiota and probiotics in production animals. *Annu. Rev. Anim. Biosci.* **2014**, *2*, 469–486. [CrossRef]
65. Fassarella, M.; Blaak, E.E.; Penders, J.; Nauta, A.; Smidt, H.; Zoetendal, E.G. Gut microbiome stability and resilience: Elucidating the response to perturbations in order to modulate gut health. *Gut* **2021**, *70*, 595–605. [CrossRef] [PubMed]
66. Marounek, M.; Březina, P.; Baran, M. Fermentation of carbohydrates and yield of microbial protein in mixed cultures of rabbit caecal microorganisms. *Arch. Anim. Nutr.* **2000**, *53*, 241–252. [CrossRef]

67. Vernay, M. Origin and utilization of volatile fatty acids and lactate in the rabbit: Influence of the faecal excretion pattern. *Br. J. Nutr.* **1987**, *57*, 371–381. [CrossRef] [PubMed]
68. De Blas, E.; Gidenne, T. Digestion of starch and sugars. In *The Nutrition of the Rabbit*; De Blas, E., Wiseman, J., Eds.; CABI Publishing: Wallingford, UK, 1998; pp. 17–38. ISBN 978-1789241273.
69. Priyadarshini, M.; Kotlo, K.U.; Dudeja, P.K.; Layden, B.T. Role of short chain fatty acid receptors in intestinal physiology and pathophysiology. *Compr. Physiol.* **2018**, *8*, 1065–1090. [CrossRef]
70. Soomro, A.H.; Masud, T.; Anwaar, K. Role of Lactic Acid Bacteria (LAB) in food preservation and human health—A review. *Pak. J. Nutr.* **2002**, *1*, 20–24.
71. Lavefve, L.; Howard, L.R.; Carbonero, F. Berry polyphenols metabolism and impact on human gut microbiota and health. *Food Funct.* **2020**, *11*, 45–65. [CrossRef] [PubMed]
72. Nardi, G.M.; De Farias Januário, A.G.; Freire, C.G.; Megiolaro, F.; Schneider, K.; Perazzoli, M.R.A.; Do Nascimento, S.R.; Gon, A.C.; Mariano, L.N.B.; Wagner, G.; et al. Anti-inflammatory activity of berry fruits in mice model of inflammation is based on oxidative stress modulation. *Pharmacogn. Res.* **2016**, *8*, S42–S49. [CrossRef]

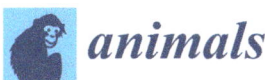

Article

# Effect of Sustained Administration of Thymol on Its Bioaccessibility and Bioavailability in Rabbits

Kristina Bacova [1,2], Karin Zitterl Eglseer [3], Gesine Karas Räuber [3], Lubica Chrastinova [4], Andrea Laukova [1], Margareta Takacsova [1], Monika Pogany Simonova [1] and Iveta Placha [1,*]

[1] Centre of Biosciences, Slovak Academy of Sciences, Institute of Animal Physiology, Soltesovej 4-6, 040 01 Kosice, Slovakia; bacovak@saske.sk (K.B.); laukova@saske.sk (A.L.); takacsova@saske.sk (M.T.); simonova@saske.sk (M.P.S.)
[2] University of Veterinary Medicine and Pharmacy, Komenskeho 73, 041 81 Kosice, Slovakia
[3] Institute of Animal Nutrition and Functional Plant Compounds, University of Veterinary Medicine Vienna, Veterinärplatz 1, A-1210 Wien, Austria; karin.zitterl@vetmeduni.ac.at (K.Z.E.); raeuber.gesine@gmail.com (G.K.R.)
[4] National Agricultural and Food Centre, Hlohovecka 2, 951 41 Nitra-Lužianky, Slovakia; lubica.chrastinova@nppc.sk
* Correspondence: placha@saske.sk; Tel.: +421-55-792-2969

**Citation:** Bacova, K.; Eglseer, K.Z.; Räuber, G.K.; Chrastinova, L.; Laukova, A.; Takacsova, M.; Simonova, M.P.; Placha, I. Effect of Sustained Administration of Thymol on Its Bioaccessibility and Bioavailability in Rabbits. *Animals* **2021**, *11*, 2595. https://doi.org/10.3390/ani11092595

Academic Editors: Alessandro Dal Bosco and Cesare Castellini

Received: 3 August 2021
Accepted: 1 September 2021
Published: 3 September 2021

**Publisher's Note:** MDPI stays neutral with regard to jurisdictional claims in published maps and institutional affiliations.

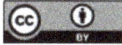

**Copyright:** © 2021 by the authors. Licensee MDPI, Basel, Switzerland. This article is an open access article distributed under the terms and conditions of the Creative Commons Attribution (CC BY) license (https://creativecommons.org/licenses/by/4.0/).

**Simple Summary:** The purpose of this study was to investigate the bioavailability and metabolic path of thymol, a major constituent of *Thymus vulgaris* L., in the rabbit organism. Oral bioavailability is a key parameter affecting the efficacy of substances, but it is not surprising that it does not correlate satisfactorily with efficacy. The main limitation factors are rate of absorption, metabolism, and excretion processes. In this work, the thymol metabolic path in the rabbit organism was determined for the first time after its sustained oral administration. We confirm intensive absorption of thymol from the gastrointestinal tract; our results point to metabolism and accumulation in kidney tissue and intensive metabolic and excretion processes in the liver. Some metabolic processes were present also after thymol withdrawal. Thymol as a lipophilic substance was found only in trace amounts in fat and muscle tissue as a consequence of its conversion into hydrophilic metabolite and greater elimination in the rabbit organism. This paper highlights the insufficient knowledge of modes of action of plant compounds in animal organisms.

**Abstract:** The objective of this study was the detection of thymol in rabbit plasma, tissues, large intestinal content, and faeces. Forty-eight rabbits were divided into control and experimental groups (thymol 250 mg/kg feed). Thymol was administered for 21 days and then withdrawn for 7 days. Concentration of thymol in the intestinal wall (IW) was significantly higher than in plasma ($p < 0.05$) and liver ($p < 0.05$); in the kidneys it was significantly higher than in plasma ($p < 0.05$) and liver ($p < 0.05$) during thymol addition. Thymol in IW was significantly higher than in plasma also after withdrawal ($p < 0.01$). Significant correlation ($r_s = -1.000$, $p < 0.01$) between IW and plasma points to the intensive absorption of thymol from the intestine, while the correlation between plasma and liver ($r_s = 0.786$, $p < 0.05$) indicates intensive biotransformation and excretion processes in liver. Significant correlation between liver and kidney ($r_s = 0.738$, $p < 0.05$) confirms the intensive metabolism of thymol in the kidney. During the withdrawal period, thymol was detected above trace amounts only in faeces, and was significantly higher than in the colon during both periods ($p < 0.01$). Results show intensive biotransformation of thymol in the rabbit organism.

**Keywords:** rabbit; thymol; absorption; distribution; accumulation; excretion

## 1. Introduction

In recent years, natural products have assumed great importance as antibiotic replacement additives and as growth promoting agents in food animals. There is large pressure on the animal production industry to improve animal treatment as well as production performance, and to ensure the safety of products for human consumption while minimizing economic losses [1]. Even though, the benefits of herbal additives depend on the biological activities of their compounds and their pharmacokinetics, their precise mode of action at the molecular level has not yet been fully elucidated [2,3].

To our knowledge, bioaccessibility, bioavailability, and metabolism of phenolic compounds have been studied in vitro in humans [4,5] and in chickens [6]. No information is available about absorption, distribution, and deposition of natural compounds at target sites in the rabbit organism. The rabbit gastrointestinal tract has characteristic features compared with other animal species, such as the relative importance of the well-developed caecum, and a separation mechanism within the proximal colon [7]. The efficiency of the rabbit's digestion depends in large part on the production and ingestion of caecotrophes, which must be considered as an integral part of the rabbit´s digestion system. The process of caecotrophy may be considered as "pseudorumination" which improves feed utilization [8,9].

One of the crucial aspects of the beneficial effect of natural compounds is the amount present in the gut as a result of their release from feed, and their consequent ability to pass through the intestinal barrier. Intestinal absorption of many compounds is limited by a range of biological and physiological barriers in the gastrointestinal tract. Biological barriers are represented mainly by the mucus layer and epithelial cell layer, which is composed of villus and crypt cells. Physiological factors include enzymatic activities in the intestinal lumen, specific transport mechanisms which are able to limit absorption, and intestinal transit time [10].

In terms of the potential role of thymol as feed additive for animals, the aim of our study was to try to produce a more detailed view and better understanding of the mechanism of its absorption, distribution, and accumulation in the rabbit organism after its sustained application into the rabbit's diet.

## 2. Materials and Methods

### 2.1. Animals Care and Use

The trial was carried out at the experimental rabbit facility of the National Agricultural and Food Centre, Research Institute for Animal Production, Nitra, Slovakia. The protocol was approved by the Institutional Ethical Committee, and the State Veterinary and Food Office of the Slovak Republic approved the experimental protocol (4047/16-221).

### 2.2. Animals and Housing

After weaning at 35 days of age, 48 rabbits of both sexes (meat line M9) were randomly divided into a control group (CG) fed a standard diet and an experimental group (EG) fed a standard diet into which 250 mg/kg of thymol was incorporated in powder form ($\geq$99.9%, Sigma-Aldrich, St. Louis, USA). All experimental wire-net cages (61 cm $\times$ 34 cm $\times$ 33 cm) were kept in rooms with automatic temperature control (22 $\pm$ 4 °C) and photoperiod (16L:8D). The rabbits could feed ad libitum and had free access to drinking water. The experiment lasted 28 days. The rabbits received feed with thymol addition for 21 days (56 d of age) and for the next 7 days (63 d of age) the thymol was withdrawn. Initial live weight was 1006 $\pm$ 98 g in CG and 1035 $\pm$ 107 g in EG (2044 $\pm$ 24 g in CG, 1965 $\pm$ 58.7 g in EG at 56 d of age, and 2671 $\pm$ 72 g in CG, 2796 $\pm$ 60 g in EG at 63 d of age). Eight rabbits in each group were killed at 56 or 63 d of age using electronarcosis (50 Hz, 0.3A/rabbit for 5 s), immediately hung by the hind legs on the processing line and quickly bled by cutting the jugular veins and the carotid arteries.

### 2.3. Diet and Chemical Analyses

The standard diet consisted of a commercial diet for growing rabbits (KKZK, Liaharensky podnik Nitra a.s., Nitra, Slovakia) with ingredients and chemical composition as shown in Table 1. The diet was administered in the form of pellets with an average size of 3.5 mm. The feed was stored in darkness to protect against degradation processes. The Association of Official Analytical Chemists (AOAC) methods [11] were used to determine the proportions of crude protein (no. 990.03, CP), ash (no. 942.05), and dry matter (no. 967.03, DM) in the diet, while DM amount was also determined for the tissues, gut content, and faeces. Neutral detergent fibre (NDF) and acid detergent fibre (ADF) were analysed according to Van Soest et al. [12].

Table 1. Ingredients (%) and chemical composition (g/kg feed) of experimental diet.

| Ingredients (%) | | Chemical Composition (g/kg Feed) | |
|---|---|---|---|
| Dehydrated lucerne meal | 36.0 | Dry matter (g/kg) | 900.9 |
| Dry malting sprouts | 15.0 | Organic compounds | 831.8 |
| Oats | 13.0 | Nitrogen free extract | 444.3 |
| Wheat bran | 9.0 | Neutral detergent fibre (NDF) | 352.9 |
| Barley | 8.0 | Acid detergent fibre (ADF) | 208.1 |
| Extracted sunflower meal | 5.5 | Crude fibre | 177.8 |
| Extracted rapeseed meal | 5.5 | Crude protein | 176.6 |
| Dried distiller grains with solubles | 5.0 | Cellulose | 163.1 |
| Premix [1] | 1.7 | Hemicellulose | 144.8 |
| Limestone | 1.0 | Starch | 133.1 |
| Sodium chloride | 0.3 | Ash | 69.2 |
| | | Fat | 33.1 |
| | | Metabolic energy, MJ/kg | 9.9 |

[1] The vitamin-mineral premix provided per kg of complete diet: Retinyl acetate 5.16 mg, Cholecalciferol 0.03 mg, Tocopherol 0.03 mg, Thiamin 0.8 mg, Riboflavin 3.0 mg, Pyridoxin 2.0 mg, Cyanocobalamin 0.02 mg, Niacin 38 mg, Folic acid 0.6 mg, Calcium 1.8 mg, Iron 70 mg, Zinc 66 mg, Copper 15, Selenium 0.25 mg.

*2.4. Thymol Stability in Feed*

Thymol evaporation in feed was analysed every week during thymol application using high-performance liquid chromatography (HPLC) according to the modified method of Oceľová [6] and Pisarčíková et al. [13]. Samples were analysed in triplicate. Briefly, 2 mL of methanol was added into a glass tube containing 0.2 g of milled feed and thymol was extracted in an ultrasonic bath. The methanolic extract was then analysed using the HPLC method with an Ultimate 3000 HPLC-system liquid chromatograph (Dionex, Sunnyvale, CA, USA). The chromatographic analyses were evaluated by means of Chromeleon® Software Version 6.80 SR10 Build 2906 (Thermo Fisher Scientific, Waltham, MA, USA).

*2.5. Sampling*

To determine the thymol content in plasma, blood (1.5 mL) from eight rabbits was collected from the marginal ear vein (*vena auricularis*) into heparinized Eppendorf tubes and plasma was obtained after centrifugation at $1180\times g$ for 15 min. The gastrointestinal tract was removed from the body cavity and was divided into small intestine, caecum, and colon (n = 8). Caecum and colon content were removed, and the small intestinal lumen was gently washed with 0.9% NaCl solution. Obtained samples of gut content and intestinal wall together with plasma, liver, kidney, muscle (*musculus longissimus dorsi*) and spleen tissue, fat, and faeces were immediately frozen in liquid nitrogen and stored at $-70\ ^\circ$C until analysis. All samples were collected at both experimental days (56 or 63 d of age).

*2.6. Thymol Analyses in Plasma, Tissues, Large Intestinal Content and Faeces*

Detection of thymol in samples of plasma, tissues and faeces was performed using headspace solid-phase microextraction followed by gas chromatography coupled with the mass spectrometry method as described by Bacova et al. [14] and Placha et al. [15]. Briefly, detection and quantification were carried out using a GC/MS (type HP 6890 GC) system coupled with a 5972-quadrupole mass-selective detector (Agilent Technologies GmbH, Wilmington, DE, USA). Detection of thymol was confirmed by comparing its specific mass spectrum and retention time with those of the reference compound. Additionally, the Kovats index was calculated. Calibration curves were generated by plotting the peak-area ratios of thymol to o-cresol used as an internal standard (Sigma-Aldrich, St Louis, MO, USA) against the known thymol concentrations. The selective ion mode was used for quantitative analysis of thymol. The mass fragments m/z 135 and m/z 150, as well as m/z 107 and m/z 108, were monitored as characteristic for thymol and o-cresol, respectively. Calibration curves were prepared from blank samples spiked directly with 50 µL thymol (Applichem, Darmstadt, Germany) in standard solutions with known concentrations as follows: for plasma 48, 100, 200, 400, and 800 ng of thymol per mL, for intestinal wall 100, 200, 400, 800, 1000 ng; for liver, kidney, muscle, caecum and colon content 100, 200, 400, 800, 1000, 2000 ng; spleen, fat 24, 50, 100, 200, 400 ng; faeces 200, 400, 800, 1600, 2000, 4000 ng of thymol per g of tissue. Each point on the calibration curve was analysed as a duplicate. The peak of thymol was detected around 19 min and the o-cresol peak occurred around 10 min in all samples. Samples for thymol detection were prepared using the method described by Oceľová et al. [16]. Enzyme β–Glucuronidase Helix pomatia Type HP-2 (aqueous solution, ≥100,000 units/mL, Sigma-Aldrich, St Louis, MO, USA) was added to samples to cleave thymol from its glucuronide and sulphate, since only free thymol should be detected in the GC system.

*2.7. Statistical Analysis*

Data collected were analysed using the Kolmogorov–Smirnov test for normal and non-normal distribution. All data were not accepted as parametric. The Kruskal–Wallis test with post hoc Dunn´s Multiple Comparison test was used to determine the differences between plasma and tissues or caecal, colon content and faeces. Results are presented as mean value ± standard error of mean (SEM). Differences were considered significant at $p < 0.05$. Correlations of thymol concentrations between plasma and intestinal wall, plasma and liver, and liver and kidney were analysed using nonparametric Spearman's Rank Correlation and expressed as Spearman's correlation coefficient ($r_s$). Statistical analyses were performed using Graph Pad Prism (GraphPad Software, San Diego, CA, USA). The experimental unit was the animal's cage.

## 3. Results

*3.1. Thymol Stability in Feed*

Concentration of thymol in feed during the period of the experiment with its addition was relatively stable at 274 µg/g DM–0 d; 255 µg/g DM–7 d; 236 µg/g DM–14 d.

*3.2. Thymol in Plasma and Tissues*

Level of thymol in the intestinal wall was significantly higher than in plasma ($p = 0.0211$) and liver ($p = 0.0305$), and in the kidneys it was significantly higher than in plasma ($p = 0.0259$) and liver ($p = 0.0415$) during the period of thymol addition (Table 2). Thymol in fat (19.9 ± 7.36 ng/g DM, n = 2) and muscle (26.6 ng/g DM, n=1) during this period was found only in a small number of samples, and only in trace amounts in others. For this reason, those samples were not included in the statistical evaluation. Significant correlation was established between thymol concentration in plasma and intestinal wall ($r_s = -1.0$, $p < 0.01$), plasma and liver ($r_s = 0.786$, $p < 0.05$) and liver and kidney ($r_s = 0.738$, $p < 0.05$, Figures 1–3). Even though thymol content was determined only in trace amounts during the period without thymol addition, the differences were statistically evaluated. Thymol in intestinal wall was significantly higher than in plasma in this period ($p = 0.0035$, Table 2).

*3.3. Thymol in Caecum, Colon and Feces*

Thymol in faeces was significantly higher than in the colon during both experimental periods, even if only in trace amounts without further thymol addition ($p < 0.01$, Table 3). During this period only thymol in faeces was detected above trace amount.

**Table 2.** Thymol content in plasma (ng/mL) and tissue (ng/g DM).

|  | 56 d of Age (with Thymol) | | 63 d of Age (without Thymol) | |
| --- | --- | --- | --- | --- |
|  | Mean | SEM | Mean | SEM |
| Plasma | 46.2 [b] | 10.0 | 2.73 [b] | 0.458 |
| Intestinal wall | 268 [a] | 65.9 | 20.4 [a] | 2.70 |
| Liver | 39.9 [b] | 13.4 | 5.93 [ab] | 0.285 |
| Kidney | 314 [a] | 91.7 | 16.1 [ab] | 6.53 |
| Spleen | 181 [ab] | 40.1 | ND | - |

[a,b] Values within a column with different superscript letters differ significantly ($p < 0.05$). Data are presented as mean ± standard error of mean (SEM).

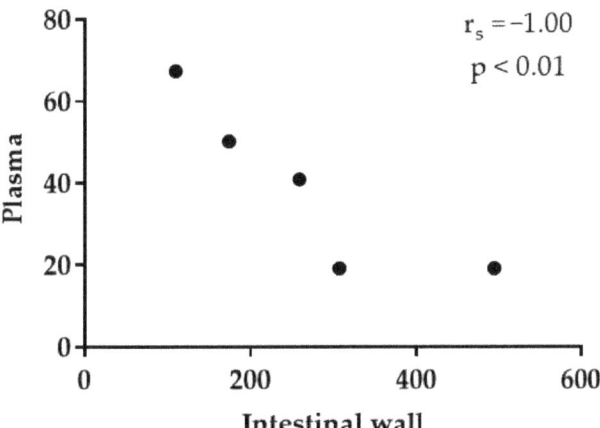

**Figure 1.** Correlation between plasma (ng/mL) and intestinal wall (ng/g DM).

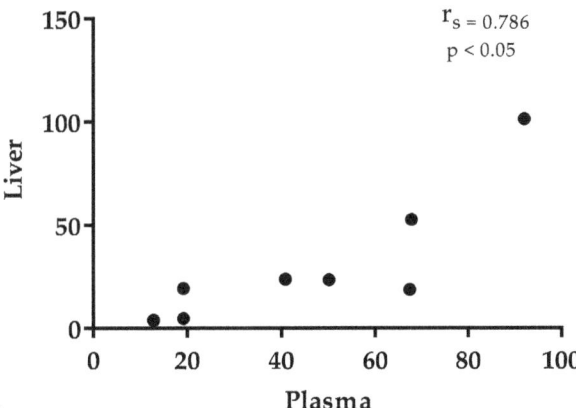

**Figure 2.** Correlation between liver (ng/g DM) and plasma (ng/mL).

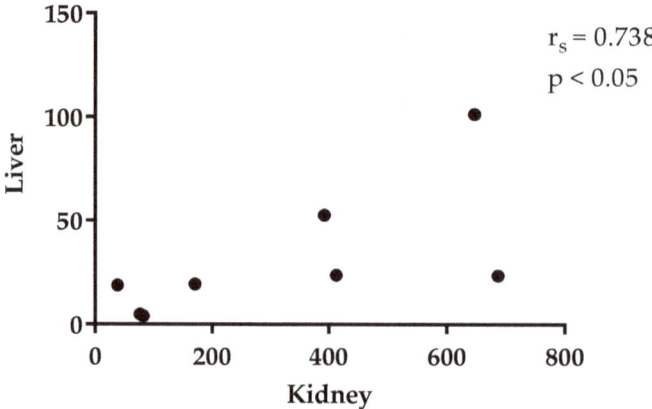

Figure 3. Correlation between liver and kidney (ng/g DM).

Table 3. Thymol content in caecum, colon, and faeces (ng/g DM).

|  | 56 d of Age (with Thymol) | | 63 d of Age (without Thymol) | |
| --- | --- | --- | --- | --- |
|  | Mean | SEM | Mean | SEM |
| Caecum | 882 [ab] | 231 | 45.8 [ab] | 12.44 |
| Colon | 672 [b] | 330 | 16.4 [b] | 9.44 |
| Faeces | 2444 [a] | 451 | 150 [a] | 40.54 |

[a,b] Values within a column with different superscript letters differ significantly ($p < 0.05$). Data are presented as mean ± standard error of mean (SEM).

## 4. Discussion

The epithelial cells in the small intestine wall contain various metabolic enzymes and transporters. The intestinal microflora possesses a wide range of metabolic processes including hydrolysis of glucuronides, sulphate esters, and amides. Enzymes in the intestinal microflora can hydrolyse drug metabolites, especially glucuronide conjugates, and convert them back to the parent compound [10]. The parent drugs excreted and/or released by the action of gut microflora are reabsorbed by intestinal cells. Metabolites are continuously excreted into the large intestine, where they are again hydrolysed and reabsorbed [17].

After being absorbed from the GIT, thymol becomes metabolized during processes of biotransformation and becomes more hydrophilic. The metabolites, mainly sulphates and glucuronides, are transported across the intestinal epithelium by active processes involving transmembrane proteins. Many transporters such as peptides, vitamins, amino acids, and sugars play important roles in the translocation of drugs and were identified in large amounts in the GIT [18].

Rubió et al. [19] and Pisarčíková et al. [13] have confirmed that thymol, which is a small lipophilic molecule, is not detected in unmetabolized form in plasma, as they detected only its conjugates (thymol sulphate and glucuronide). They also detected thymol conjugates in the duodenal wall, which points to active biotransformation of thymol in the organism.

Significant correlation ($r_s = -1.00$, $p < 0.01$) between thymol content in the intestinal wall and plasma in our experiment indicates intensive absorption of thymol from the intestine. Placha et al. [15] and Oceľová et al. [20] also confirmed the intensive absorption of thymol from all intestinal segments in broiler chickens after four weeks of diet supplementation with thyme essential oil. They found significant correlation between thymol content in plasma and individual intestinal segments. Although we found six times lower concentration of thymol in plasma during its addition and seven times lower after its withdrawal (even if only in trace amounts) in comparison with the intestinal wall, we can confirm that some metabolic processes were still active after thymol withdrawal from feed (Tables 2 and 3).

The rabbit caecum is the largest part of the large intestine and contains approximately 40% of the intestinal content. The primary mechanism by which nutrients are released from intestinal content is microbial fermentation, and its products are absorbed through the intestinal wall or are reingested as caecotrophes. The retained particles from the proximal part of the colon also provide substrate for caecal microbiota. The mucus which coats the caecotrophes protects them and allows the fermentation processes to continue in them until they reach the intestine. The composition of the intestinal flora depends to a large extent on the caecotrophic microbial population [21].

Intestinal microflora and epithelial cells play a crucial role in metabolic processes because they produce a wide range of metabolic enzymes [22]. The counts of bacterial flora are highly variable in different parts of the gastrointestinal tract [23]. We assume that the metabolic enzymes responsible for thymol biotransformation in the caecum and consequently in caecotrophes are expressed in large enough amounts that they can affect metabolic activities and consequently exert influence on the amount of thymol and its metabolites in the caecum.

There are some conditions affecting the absorption of compounds in the GIT. In addition to their rate of dissolution in the intestinal fluids, they must also be able to cross membranes in each part of the GIT. In case they are not able to cross these membranes by the time they reach the colon, the extent of intestinal absorption is not sufficient, and the compounds are excreted in faeces [24]. All these circumstances may explain the high concentrations of thymol in the caecum and faeces, not only during its addition but also after its withdrawal from feed (Table 3).

The first study which confirmed the presence of thymol metabolites (thymol sulphate and glucuronide) in the duodenal wall of broiler chickens after sustained consumption of thyme essential oil also confirmed the key role of the intestine in the metabolism of thymol [13]. Oceľová [6] detected thymol in the liver at a level of 8.9% of its concentration in the intestinal wall and observed significant correlation between thymol concentrations in liver and plasma, and liver and intestinal wall, which might indicate sufficient absorption of thymol from the intestinal wall to the liver through the vena portae. We found 15% (with thymol) and 29% (without thymol) of thymol in liver compared with its content in the intestinal wall, and significant correlation between thymol concentrations in plasma and liver ($r_s = 0.7857$, $p < 0.05$). These results are in agreement with the findings of the above-mentioned authors and point to intensive biotransformation and excretion processes in the liver.

Between the enzyme systems and efflux transporters there exist mutual processes which can affect the efficiency of drugs in the intestine. These couplings can prolong the exposure of drugs in vivo and are crucial for enteric and enterohepatic recycling. Some parent compounds are absorbed and metabolized in the intestinal cells, while some portions are effluxed back into the intestinal lumen or transported to the mesenteric vein and are taken up by hepatocytes [17]. Excreted metabolites from enterocytes are converted back to the parent compound and again reabsorbed. Compounds in the liver are metabolized and together with parent compounds are excreted with bile into the duodenum and are then reabsorbed there [14,17]. These repeating processes together with processes of caecotrophy could explain the thymol content in plasma, tissues, and intestinal content after thymol withdrawal, although only in trace amounts. We must point out that we detected the sum of metabolized and non-metabolized thymol, as the thymol metabolites were cleaved by added enzyme, β-glucuronidase. However, the extent of absorption of compounds (drugs) and the contribution to their bioavailability by metabolic enzymes and transporters or receptors present on the intestinal membrane are still not clear.

In the present study, a significantly higher level of thymol in the kidney in comparison with liver tissue and plasma confirmed its metabolism and/or accumulation in this organ (Table 2). Our results are in agreement with our previous study [6], in which we detected a significantly higher thymol concentration in the kidney of chickens with thyme essential oil diet supplementation. Takada [25] detected thymol glucuronide and thymol sulphate in the urine of rabbits, and to our knowledge this is the only study concerned with the metabolic path of thymol in these animals. Data available so far indicate that thymol sulphate could be reabsorbed in the proximal tubule after glomerulary filtration, and that cleavage of this metabolite is achieved by enzymes located at the luminal brush border, so that subsequently thymol could be reabsorbed [26]. These authors demonstrated that although the liver is the most important organ for biotransformation, kidney microsomes demonstrate more effective metabolic processes than liver or intestinal microsomes. The significantly higher content of thymol in the kidney and the correlation between liver and kidney ($r_s$ = 0.7381, $p$ < 0.05) in our study also confirm the intensive metabolism in kidney tissue. However, further study of renal metabolism mechanisms is necessary to confirm these findings.

Before drug compounds can reach systemic circulation and therapeutic targets, several barriers must be overcome [18]. Although lipophilic molecules evidently pass the barriers with ease by transcellular routes, various efflux transporters are preferentially bound with lipophilic molecules, seriously limiting their absorption. The first-pass metabolism which occurs in the intestinal wall decreases the chance of molecules which get into epithelial cells to reach the systemic circulation. Once compounds are absorbed in the GIT, the next major barrier awaits in the form of the first-pass metabolism in the liver. Drugs passing through the portal vein encounter hepatocytes and are metabolized there [18]. Based on these processes we can explain the trace amounts of thymol detected in rabbit muscle and fat in our experiment. Trace amounts of thymol in the muscle tissue of broiler chickens were also detected by Haselmeyer et al. [27] after thymol addition (55 mg/kg DM feed), and by Oceľová [6] after thyme essential oil application. Lipophilic substances which are not metabolized during the process of biotransformation are less readily eliminated and accumulate in fat tissue [22]. As we found only traces of thymol in this tissue, we can hypothesize that the majority of thymol was metabolized and converted into hydrophilic substances.

Finally, little is known about the bioactivity of thymol and thymol metabolites, further studies are needed to evaluate the distribution of thymol in different tissues at different levels and establish its suitable concentration for a beneficial effect on animal health.

## 5. Conclusions

Our results showed that, thymol was efficiently absorbed from the intestinal lumen and intensive metabolic processes in liver and kidney were observed, while accumulation in fat and muscle tissue was low, probably due to its intensive biotransformation into hydrophilic substances which were then excreted. We confirm some metabolic processes involving thymol even after its withdrawal from feed, as a consequence of caecotrophy. Oral bioavailability of plant compounds is a challenge for scientists because their metabolic processes in the animal organism should be understood at molecular level.

**Author Contributions:** Conceptualization: I.P.; methodology: I.P., K.B.; validation: I.P.; formal analysis: I.P., K.Z.E., K.B., G.K.R., M.T.; M.P.S.; investigation: I.P., K.B.; resources: I.P., K.Z.E.; data curation: I.P., L.C., A.L.; writing—original draft preparation: I.P., K.B.; writing—review and editing: K.Z.E.; visualization: I.P., K.B.; project administration: I.P.; funding acquisition: I.P. All authors have read and agreed to the published version of the manuscript.

**Funding:** This research was funded by the Scientific Grant Agency of the Ministry for Education, Science, Research and Sport of the Slovak Republic and the Slovak Academy of Sciences (VEGA 2/0009/20), as well as the Austrian Federal Ministry for Science, Research and Economics, OeAD, Ernst Mach Grant Action Austria-Slovakia.

**Institutional Review Board Statement:** The study was conducted according to the guidelines of the Declaration of Helsinki, and approved by the Ethics Committee of the State Veterinary and Food Office of the Slovak Republic on 1 December 2016 (approval number SK CH 17016).

**Data Availability Statement:** Data availability upon reasonable request to the corresponding author.

**Acknowledgments:** The authors gratefully acknowledge the technical support provided by M. Madarova at the University of Veterinary Medicine and Pharmacy, Kosice, Slovakia and L. Ondruska, V. Parkanyi and R. Jurcik at the National Agricultural and Food Centre, Research Institute for Animal Production, Nitra, Slovakia. The authors also thank Andrew Billingham for improving the written English of the manuscript.

**Conflicts of Interest:** The authors declare no conflict of interest. The funders had no role in the design of the study; in the collection, analyses, or interpretation of data; in the writing of the manuscript, or in the decision to publish the results.

## References

1. Kostadinović, L.; Lević, J. Effect of phytoadditives in poultry and pig diseases. *J. Agron. Technol. Eng. Manag.* **2018**, *1*, 1–7.
2. Diaz-Sanchez, S.; D'Souza, D.; Biswas, D.; Hanning, I. Botanical alternatives to antibiotics for use in organic poultry production. *Poult. Sci.* **2015**, *94*, 1419–1430. [CrossRef] [PubMed]
3. Gadde, U.; Kim, W.H.; Oh, S.T.; Lillehoj, H.S. Alternatives to antibiotics for maximizing growth performance and feed efficiency in poultry: A review. *Anim. Health Res. Rev.* **2017**, *18*, 26–45. [CrossRef]
4. Rubió, L.; Farràs, M.; de La Torre, R.; Macià, A.; Romero, M.P.; Valls, R.M.; Solà, R.; Farré, M.; Fitó, M.; Motilva, M.J. Metabolite profiling of olive oil and thyme phenols after a sustained intake of two phenol-enriched olive oils by humans: Identification of compliance markers. *Food Res. Int.* **2014**, *65*, 59–68. [CrossRef]
5. Rubió, L.; Macià, A.; Castell-Auví, A.; Pinent, M.; Blay, M.T.; Ardévol, A.; Romero, M.P.; Motilva, M.J. Effect of the co-occurring olive oil and thyme extracts on the phenolic bioaccessibility and bioavailability assessed by in vitro digestion and cell models. *Food Chem.* **2014**, *149*, 277–284. [CrossRef] [PubMed]
6. Ocel'ová, V. Plant Additives in Relation to the Animal Gastrointestinal Tract and Metabolism of Their Main Compounds. Ph.D Thesis, Institute of Animal Physiology, Slovak Academy of Sciences, Košice, Slovakia, 2017.
7. Sakaguchi, E. Digestive strategies of small hindgut fermenters. *Anim. Sci. J.* **2003**, *74*, 327–337. [CrossRef]
8. Hirakawa, H. Coprophagy in leporids and other mammalian herbivores. *Mammal Rev.* **2001**, *31*, 61–80. [CrossRef]
9. Irlbeck, N.A. How to feed the rabbit (Oryctolagus cuniculus) gastrointestinal tract. *J. Anim. Sci.* **2001**, *79*, E343–E346. [CrossRef]
10. Ho, P.C. Biological and physiological features of the gastrointestinal tract relevant to oral drug absorption. In *Oral Bioavailability: Basic Principles, Advanced Concepts, and Applications*; Hu, M., Li, X., Eds.; John Wiley & Sons, Inc.: Hoboken, NJ, USA, 2011; pp. 51–61.
11. Association of Official Analytical Chemists (AOAC). *International Official Methods of Analysis*, 18th ed.; AOAC: Gaithersburg, MD, USA, 2005.
12. Van Soest, P.J.; Robertson, J.B.; Lewis, B. A methods for dietary fiber, neutral detergent fiber, and nonstarch polysaccharides in relation to animal nutrition. *J. Dairy Sci.* **1991**, *74*, 3583–3597. [CrossRef]
13. Pisarčíková, J.; Ocel'ová, V.; Faix, Š.; Plachá, I.; Calderón, A.I. Identification and quantification of thymol metabolites in plasma, liver and duodenal wall of broiler chickens using UHPLC-ESI-QTOF-MS. *Biomed. Chromatogr.* **2017**, *31*, e3881. [CrossRef] [PubMed]
14. Bacova, K.; Zitterl-Eglseer, K.; Chrastinova, L.; Laukova, A.; Madarova, M.; Gancarcikova, S.; Sopkova, D.; Andrejcakova, Z.; Placha, I. Effect of thymol addition and withdrawal on some blood parameters, antioxidative defence system and fatty acid profile in rabbit muscle. *Animals* **2020**, *10*, 1248. [CrossRef] [PubMed]
15. Placha, I.; Ocelova, V.; Chizzola, R.; Battelli, G.; Gai, F.; Bacova, K.; Faix, S. Effect of thymol on the broiler chicken antioxidative defence system after sustained dietary thyme oil application. *Br. Poult. Sci.* **2019**, *60*, 589–596. [CrossRef] [PubMed]
16. Ocel'ová, V.; Chizzola, R.; Pisarčíková, J.; Novak, J.; Ivanišinová, O.; Faix, Š. Effect of thyme essential oil supplementation on thymol content in blood plasma, liver, kidney and muscle in broiler chickens. *Nat. Prod. Commun.* **2016**, *11*, 1545–1550. [CrossRef] [PubMed]
17. Singh, R.; Hu, M. Drug metabolism in gastroinestinal tract. In *Oral Bioavailability: Basic Principles, Advanced Concepts, and Applications*; Hu, M., Li, X., Eds.; John Wiley & Sons, Inc.: Hoboken, NJ, USA, 2011; pp. 91–109.
18. Hu, M.; Li, X. Barriers to oral bioavailability-an overview. In *Oral Bioavailability: Basic Principles, Advanced Concepts, and Applications*; Hu, M., Li, X., Eds.; John Wiley & Sons, Inc.: Hoboken, NJ, USA, 2011; pp. 1–5.
19. Rubió, L.; Serra, A.; Macià, A.; Borràs, X.; Romero, M.P.; Motilva, M.J. Validation of determination of plasma metabolites derived from thyme bioactive compounds by improved liquid chromatography coupled to tandem mass spectrometry. *J. Chromatogr. B* **2012**, *905*, 75–84. [CrossRef] [PubMed]
20. Ocel'ová, V.; Chizzola, R.; Battelli, G.; Pisarcikova, J.; Faix, S.; Gai, F.; Placha, I. Thymol in the intestinal tract of broiler chickens after sustained administration of thyme essential oil in feed. *J. Anim. Physiol. Anim. Nutr.* **2018**, *103*, 204–209. [CrossRef] [PubMed]
21. Campbell-Ward, M.L. Gastrointestinal physiology and nutrition. In *Ferrets, Rabbits, and Rodents: Clinical Medicine and Surgery*, 3rd ed.; Quesenberry, K.E., Carpenter, J.W., Eds.; Elsevier: Saint-Louis, MO, USA, 2012; pp. 183–192.
22. Skálová, L.; Boušová, I. *Metabolismus Léčivých a Jiných Xenobiotik*; Karolinum: Praha, Czech Republic, 2011; p. 162.

23. Ding, X.; Kaminsky, L.S. Human extrahepatic cytochromes P450: Function in xenobiotic metabolism and tissue-selective chemical toxicity in the respiratory and gastrointestinal tracts. *Annu. Rev. Pharmacol. Toxicol.* **2003**, *43*, 149–173. [CrossRef] [PubMed]
24. Park, M.S.; Chang, J.H. Absorption of drugs via passive diffusion and carrier-mediated pathways. In *Oral Bioavailability: Basic Principles, Advanced Concepts, and Applications*; Hu, M., Li, X., Eds.; John Wiley & Sons, Inc.: Hoboken, NJ, USA, 2011; pp. 63–75.
25. Takada, M.; Agata, I.; Sakamoto, M.; Yagi, N.; Hayashi, N. On the metabolic detoxication of thymol in rabbit and man. *J. Toxicol. Sci.* **1979**, *4*, 341–350. [CrossRef] [PubMed]
26. Kohlert, C.; Schindler, G.; März, R.W.; Abel, G.; Brinkhaus, B.; Derendorf, H.; Gräfe, E.U.; Veit, M. Systemic availability and pharmacokinetics of thymol in humans. *J. Clin. Pharmacol.* **2002**, *42*, 731–737. [CrossRef]
27. Haselmeyer, A.; Zentek, J.; Chizzola, R. Effects of thyme as a feed additive in broiler chickens on thymol in gut contents, blood plasma, liver and muscle. *J. Sci. Food Agric.* **2015**, *95*, 504–508. [CrossRef]

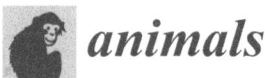

Article

# Effect of Goji Berry (*Lycium barbarum*) Supplementation on Reproductive Performance of Rabbit Does

Egon Andoni [1,†], Giulio Curone [2,†], Stella Agradi [2], Olimpia Barbato [3], Laura Menchetti [4,*], Daniele Vigo [2], Riccardo Zelli [3], Elisa Cotozzolo [5], Maria Rachele Ceccarini [6], Massimo Faustini [2], Alda Quattrone [3], Marta Castrica [7] and Gabriele Brecchia [2]

1. Faculty of Veterinary Medicine, Agricultural University of Albania, 1029 Kamez, Albania; eandoni@ubt.edu.al
2. Department of Veterinary Medicine, University of Milano, 26900 Lodi, Italy; giulio.curone@unimi.it (G.C.); stella.agradi@unimi.it (S.A.); daniele.vigo@unimi.it (D.V.); massimo.faustini@unimi.it (M.F.); gabriele.brecchia@unimi.it (G.B.)
3. Department of Veterinary Medicine, University of Perugia, 06121 Perugia, Italy; olimpia.barbato@unipg.it (O.B.); riccardo.zelli@unipg.it (R.Z.); alda.quattrone@hotmail.it (A.Q.)
4. Department of Agricultural and Food Sciences, University of Bologna, 40137 Bologna, Italy
5. Department of Agricultural, Food and Environmental Sciences, University of Perugia, 06121 Perugia, Italy; elisa.cotozzolo@studenti.unipg.it
6. Department of Pharmaceutical Sciences, University of Perugia, 06123 Perugia, Italy; mariarachele.ceccarini@unipg.it
7. Department of Health, Animal Science and Food Safety "Carlo Cantoni", University of Milano, 20133 Milan, Italy; marta.castrica@unimi.it
* Correspondence: laura.menchetti7@gmail.com; Tel.: +39-02-503-34583
† These authors contribute equally to this work.

**Simple Summary:** Infectious diseases represent serious problems for the reproductive performance of livestock animals because they negatively affect not only the welfare of the animals, but also the profitability of the farm. Moreover, the European Community continues to promote the reduction of the use of antibiotics and hormones in animal breeding. In this context, it is necessary to find new nutritional approaches to reduce the negative energy balance, and at the same time, to reinforce the immune system of the animals. In this research, the effect of goji berry supplementation on the reproductive activity and productive performance of rabbits is evaluated. *Lycium barbarum* fruit is considered a nutraceutical natural product containing various biologically active substances that show health benefits for both humans and animals. In particular, the berry can modulate hormones and metabolites involved in energy balance and reproduction, stimulate and balance the immune system activity, contributing to the defense of the organism against pathogens. Our results suggest that the integration with goji berry in the rabbit diet at 1% affects the reproductive activity, influencing the pattern secretion of luteinizing hormone (LH) and estrogens, as well as the sexual receptivity. Moreover, the fruit induced a higher milk production, improving the productive performance of young rabbits.

**Abstract:** Goji berry shows a wide range of beneficial properties in human health, but only a few studies evaluated its effects in livestock animals. The objective of this research was to assess the effects of goji berry supplementation on the hormonal profile, productive, and reproductive performance of does. Two months before artificial insemination, 105 nulliparous does were randomly divided into three groups ($n = 35$) based on the dietary treatment: commercial diet (C), or a diet supplemented with either 1% (G1), or 3% (G3) of goji berry, respectively. The results showed that receptivity was higher in G1 than in the C group ($p < 0.05$). Trends toward significance for differences between the G1 and G3 groups in marginal means of LH concentrations ($p = 0.059$), and between G1 and C in LH AUC values ($p = 0.078$), were evidenced. Estrogen concentrations showed a more fluctuating trend but a significant interaction effect ($p < 0.001$). The G1 group showed higher litter weight than C at birth ($p = 0.008$) and weaning ($p < 0.001$), as well as higher litter size at weaning ($p = 0.020$). The G1 group also exhibited the highest mean milk production ($p < 0.01$). In conclusion, goji berry influenced

Citation: Andoni, E.; Curone, G.; Agradi, S.; Barbato, O.; Menchetti, L.; Vigo, D.; Zelli, R.; Cotozzolo, E.; Ceccarini, M.R.; Faustini, M.; et al. Effect of Goji Berry (*Lycium barbarum*) Supplementation on Reproductive Performance of Rabbit Does. *Animals* **2021**, *11*, 1672. https://doi.org/10.3390/ani11061672

Academic Editors: Iveta Plachá, Monika Pogány Simonová and Andrea Lauková

Received: 12 May 2021
Accepted: 1 June 2021
Published: 3 June 2021

**Publisher's Note:** MDPI stays neutral with regard to jurisdictional claims in published maps and institutional affiliations.

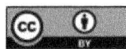

Copyright: © 2021 by the authors. Licensee MDPI, Basel, Switzerland. This article is an open access article distributed under the terms and conditions of the Creative Commons Attribution (CC BY) license (https://creativecommons.org/licenses/by/4.0/).

reproductive and productive performance, probably via modulating hormonal patterns and milk production in rabbits. However, further studies are needed to validate these preliminary results.

**Keywords:** receptivity; fertility; estrogen; LH; milk production

## 1. Introduction

*Lycium barbarum*, also known as wolfberry or Goji berry, is a functional food and plant medicine that has been used in China and Asian countries for 2300 years to restore well-being, improve eyesight, and nourish the kidneys and liver [1]. Recent studies have shown that goji berries possess various benefits for human health such as anti-aging [2], antioxidant [3], antidiabetic [4], hypolipidaemic [5], anticancer [6], cytoprotective [7], neuroprotective [8,9], immunomodulatory [10], gastroprotective [11], radiation protecting [12], and visual protecting effects [13]. As a consequence of all these beneficial properties and of the increasing public awareness of health and the quality of life, the plant and the fruit of *Lycium barbarum* have become extraordinarily popular in Western countries, where its cultivation and consumption have increased [1]. Moreover, the fruit seems to have a high safety profile at different dosages [14], although a few studies reported mild toxicity [15] and adverse effects such as urticarial-like reactions related to its use [16]. Goji berry contains a high quantity of carbohydrates, dietary fiber, protein, macro and micronutrients, and low levels of fat [17]. Besides the high nutritional value, it contains many biologically active compounds such as polysaccharides, carotenoids, phenylpropanoids, phenolics, and flavonoids [18]. Several studies showed that the wide range of effects of goji berries are principally due to the biological properties of polysaccharides [1]. They represent the most abundant constituents of the fresh and dried berry (46–51% and 5–8%, respectively), and are found principally branched and in the water-soluble form [14].

The research activity concerning goji berries was mainly carried out on humans, laboratory animals, and on specific cell lines in vitro [4,9,10,19], while only a few investigations have been carried out on livestock animals [20], including rabbits [21–23]. The rabbit is considered a livestock animal, and the productive efficiency of rabbit farms is strongly influenced by reproductive performance, especially those of the rabbit does. Generally, nulliparous does show higher fertility than primiparous and multiparous does [24,25]. The major causes of the reduced fertility rate of primiparous does are both the intensive reproductive rhythms to which they are subjected, and the negative energy balance due to the overlap between pregnancy and lactation [26,27]. Moreover, the profitability of the breeders could be reduced by the high culling and mortality rate of the animals, and the costs related to the purchase of medicines and veterinary services as a consequence of the sanitary status of the farm. Poor hygiene and incorrect artificial insemination practices are often linked to the onset of clinical or subclinical endometritis and metritis, which reduce the reproductive performance of the does [28,29]. Local and systemic diseases and/or inflammatory status induce the release of chemokines by the activation of TLR4 receptors that mobilize and activate immune cells [30]. At the systemic level, an alteration of the hormonal secretion of the gonadal axis could be induced; whereas at a local level, the inflammatory mediators and other signaling molecules can influence cellular, vascular, and endocrine functions impairing the reproductive activity of the animals [31,32].

Infectious diseases are generally fought with antibiotics, yet in the last decade, the abuse of these drugs led to the onset of antibiotic resistance with a dangerous and direct impact on human and animal health [33,34]. For this reason, the European Community guidelines tend to reduce the use of antibiotics and hormones in animal husbandry, including rabbit farming [35]. In this context, there has been a growing interest in the study and research of nutraceutical products that show health-promoting effects and with a potential in the prevention and treatment of several human and animal diseases, including those of the reproductive system [36,37]. Although there are numerous studies on the biological activity of goji berries, their effects on the reproductive functions, gonadic axis activity, and fertility, are poorly known [38,39]. In particular, the research is strongly limited for the female of both humans and animals, including rabbit does [40,41]. The rabbit is, however, an excellent animal model for research, in particular with regards to the physiology of reproduction and several reproductive parameters [42–44].

Goji berry could be a natural strategy to improve the reproductive performance of rabbit farms. It is speculated that the fruit could reduce the incidence of reproductive infections/inflammation of the genital tract, acting principally on the immune system and the oxidative status of the organs as well as influencing the hormonal secretion of the ovarian axis. Therefore, the main objective of the present study is to evaluate the effect of goji berry dietary supplementation on the reproductive performance, fertility, LH, and estrogen secretion, as well as the milk production, of rabbit does.

## 2. Materials and Methods

### 2.1. Animals and Experimental Design

The experiment was conducted at the farm of the Agricultural University of Tirana, Faculty of Veterinary Medicine, Albania. The animals were maintained in accordance with Legislative Decree No. 146, implementing Directive 98/58/EC regarding the protection of animals that were kept for farming purposes. The experimental protocol was run with the permission of the Ministry of Agriculture and Rural Development, National Authority of Veterinary and Plants protection (prot. 824/2020), of Albania. All efforts were made to minimize animal distress and to use only the number of animals necessary to produce reliable results. Moreover, the responsible veterinarian for the farm checked the rabbits for health and welfare states daily.

Nulliparous New Zealand White rabbits ($n$ = 105) of 4 months of age, weighing 3.5–3.8 kg, were individually housed in controlled environmental conditions where the temperature ranged from +18 to +21 °C, the relative humidity from 55% to 65%, the artificial ventilation was 0.3 m$^3$/s, and the lighting was scheduled 16 L:8 D at 40 lux. Rabbits were provided 150 g/d of commercial food and water ad libitum. The composition of the diet supplied to the does is described in Table 1 and is in agreement with previous studies [21–23]. Goji berries in dried form were provided by a farm of central Italy (Impresa Agricola Gianluca Bazzica, Foligno, Italy). They were ground into smaller pieces, mixed with the rest of the diet ingredients, and, finally, pelleted [23]. All rabbits completely consumed their daily rations.

**Table 1.** Formulation and chemical composition (as fed) of control (C) and experimental diets supplemented with 1% (G1) and 3% (G3) Goji berries.

| Ingredients/Analytical Data | Diet | | |
| --- | --- | --- | --- |
| | C | G1 | G3 |
| **Ingredients** [1] | | | |
| Wheat bran | 30.0 | 29.5 | 29.0 |
| Dehydrated alfalfa meal | 42.0 | 41.5 | 41.0 |
| Barley | 9.5 | 9.5 | 9.0 |
| Sunflower meal | 4.5 | 4.5 | 4.2 |
| Rice bran | 4.0 | 4.0 | 3.9 |
| Soybean meal | 4.0 | 4.0 | 3.9 |
| Calcium carbonate | 2.2 | 2.2 | 2.2 |
| Cane molasses | 2.0 | 2.0 | 2.0 |
| Dicalcium phosphate | 0.7 | 0.7 | 0.7 |
| Vitamin-mineral premix [2] | 0.4 | 0.4 | 0.4 |
| Soybean oil | 0.4 | 0.4 | 0.4 |
| Salt | 0.3 | 0.3 | 0.3 |
| Goji berries | - | 1.0 | 3.0 |

Table 1. Cont.

| Ingredients/Analytical Data | Diet | | |
| --- | --- | --- | --- |
| | C | G1 | G3 |
| Analytical data [1] | | | |
| Crude Protein | 15.74 | 15.64 | 15.66 |
| Ether extract | 2.25 | 2.23 | 2.47 |
| Ash | 9.28 | 9.36 | 9.25 |
| Starch | 16.86 | 17.07 | 16.99 |
| NDF | 38.05 | 38.55 | 37.49 |
| ADF | 19.54 | 19.60 | 19.01 |
| ADL | 4.01 | 4.31 | 3.98 |
| Digestible Energy [3] | 2464 | 2463 | 2459 |

[1] as percentage (%). [2] Per kg diet: vitamin A 11,000 IU; vitamin D3 2000 IU; vitamin B1 2.5 mg; vitamin B2 4 mg; vitamin B6 1.25 mg; vitamin B12 0.01 mg; alpha-tocopherol acetate 50 mg; biotine 0.06 mg; vitamin K 2.5 mg; niacin 15 mg; folic acid 0.30 mg; D-pantothenic acid 10 mg; choline 600 mg; Mn 60 mg; Fe 50 mg; Zn 15 mg; I 0.5 mg; Co 0.5 mg. [3] as Kcal/kg. Estimated by Maertens et al. [45].

The does were randomly divided into three different groups ($n$ = 35/group), according to the dietary treatment: commercial diet (Control, C), and diet supplemented with 1% or 3% of goji berry, G1 and G3 groups, respectively. After a period of adaptation to the new feed for two months, the does were submitted to artificial insemination (AI) at 6 months of age, performed with a heterospermic pool of fresh semen (0.5 mL) diluted 1:5 in a commercial extender. At the moment of the insemination, receptivity was established by controlling for the color of the vulva, and ovulation was induced by an intramuscular injection of 10 µg of synthetic gonadotropin-releasing hormone (GnRH; Receptal, Hoechst-Roussel Vet, Milan, Italy) [31]. Day 0 was designed as the day of the insemination. Pregnancy was diagnosed by abdominal palpation 12 days after AI, and then, 25 pregnant rabbit does per group were followed until the weaning of the young rabbits (day 35). Lactation was controlled by opening the door of the nest one time a day until 18 days after parturition.

On the day of the AI, blood samples were collected every 60 minutes, starting 120 minutes before and up to 240 minutes after the AI and GnRH injection to evaluate LH and 17-β estradiol concentrations. The samples were withdrawn from the marginal ear vein by a butterfly needle of 24G connected to a syringe of 2.5 mL. Blood samples were inserted into tubes containing EDTA, and immediately centrifuged at 3000× $g$ for 15 min; furthermore, plasma was stored frozen until it was assayed for hormone levels.

The following reproductive and productive indices were calculated: receptivity (color of the vulva [46] categorized as white, pink, or red), fertility (number of parturitions/number of inseminations × 100), milk production, litter weight (from delivery until day 18 of the whole litter, and from day 18 to weaning of the single animal), litter size, and pre-weaning mortality (calculated as the percentage of weaned kits/litter) [47]. From parturition to day 35, the mortality, the litter weight, and the litter size were recorded daily. Milk production was evaluated daily by weighing the does before and after suckling, from parturition until day 18 of lactation [48].

### 2.2. Hormone and Metabolite Assays

Plasma LH concentrations were evaluated using a commercial rabbit LH ELISA kit (Wuhan Fine Biotech Co., Ltd., Wuhan, Hubei, China). The determination procedure is based on a sandwich enzyme-linked immune-sorbent assay technology. The kit shows high sensitivity, with a limit of detection of 0.281 ng/mL and excellent specificity for the detection of LH. The intra- and inter-assay coefficients of variation were <8 and <10%, respectively. Values below and above the limits of detection of the test were considered to be 0 and 30 ng / mL, respectively.

Plasma 17β-oestradiol concentrations in plasma samples were assayed using a commercial RIA kit (Immunotech sro, Prague, Czech Republic) following the procedure indicated by the producer [49]. The limit of detection was 13,11 pg/ml and the intra- and inter-assay coefficients of variation were <14.4 and <14.5%, respectively. Values below the limit of detection of the test were considered to be 0 pg/mL.

## 2.3. Statistical Analysis

Kolmogorov-Smirnov and Levene tests were used to verify assumptions. Hormone concentrations and milk yield were analyzed by mixed-design ANOVA followed by multiple comparison tests corrected using the Bonferroni–Sidak method. Mixed design ANOVA evaluated the effect of dietary treatment (i.e., group effect; 3 levels: C, G1, and G3 groups), change over time (i.e., repeated-measures effect; 7 levels for hormone concentrations and 18 levels for milk yield), and their interaction. The LH AUC (area under the curve) was calculated for each animal by the trapezoid method using LH values at each sampling time point from 0 to 240 from the GnRH injection [48,50]. LH AUC, litter size, and weights were compared between groups by one-way ANOVA. Finally, receptivity and fertility were analyzed by Chi-square tests to evaluate if there was an association between these parameters and dietary treatment. The proportions of each group were then compared by pairwise z-tests. Statistical analyses were performed with SPSS Statistics version 25 (IBM, SPSS Inc., Chicago, IL, USA) and GraphPad Prism version 5.01 software (Inc., San Diego, CA, USA). We defined $p \leq 0.05$ as significant and $p < 0.1$ as a trend.

## 3. Results

### 3.1. Hormone Concentrations

Regardless of the group, plasma LH levels reached a peak at 60–120 minutes after GnRH injection (20.3 ± 1.1 ng/ml and 15.8 ± 2.2 ng/ml at 60 and 120 min, respectively; $p$ for time effect <0.0001) and returned to baseline levels after 240 minutes (Figure 1). Regarding the group effect, trends toward significance were found for both LH concentrations ($p = 0.056$) and LH AUC ($p = 0.067$). In particular, multiple comparisons showed that marginal means of LH concentrations tended to be higher in G1 than in G3 (7.9 ± 3.2 and 6.5 ± 3.1 ng/ml for G1 and G3, respectively; $p = 0.059$), while LH AUC tended to be higher in G1 than in C (2510 ± 175 ng/ml x h and 3031 ± 149 ng/ml x h for C and G1, respectively; $p = 0.078$).

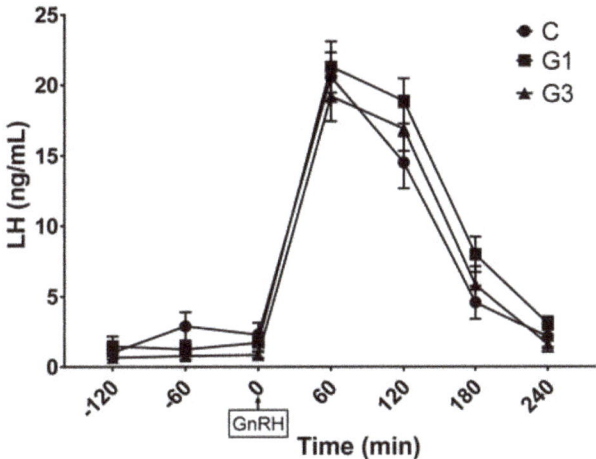

**Figure 1.** Plasma luteinizing hormone (LH) concentrations from minutes −120 to 240 after GnRH injection in the control group (C) and does supplemented with 1% (G1) or 3% (G3) of Goji. Values are means and standard errors.

Estrogen concentrations showed a more fluctuating trend, even if the highest mean values, regardless of group, were found at 180 minutes after GnRH injection ($p$ for time effect <0.0001; Figure 2). Estrogen concentrations also showed a significant interaction effect ($p < 0.001$) and a trend toward significance for a group effect ($p = 0.065$). In particular, marginal means of the G1 group tended to be higher than in C (6.2 ± 1.9 pg/mL and 8.5 ± 3.0 pg/mL for C and G1, respectively; $p = 0.088$), and multiple comparisons showed significant differences between groups at time 0 ($p = 0.034$). Moreover, rabbits of the G3 group showed a delayed estrogen peak compared to the other two groups.

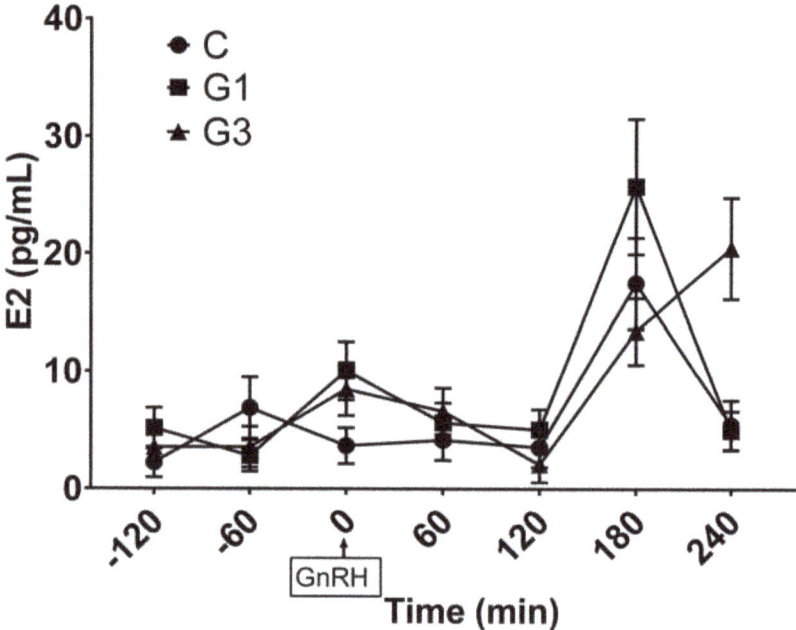

**Figure 2.** Plasma estrogen (E2) concentrations from minutes −120 to 240 after GnRH injection in the control group (C) and does supplemented with 1% (G1) or 3% (G3) of Goji. Values are means and standard errors.

*3.2. Reproductive and Productive Performance*

As an indicator of a rabbit doe's receptivity, the color of the vulva was affected by nutritional treatment ($p = 0.044$). In particular, the percentage of does showing a white color of the vulva was lower in G1 than in the C group, while the percentage of does showing a red color was higher in G1 than in the G3 group ($p < 0.05$; Figure 3). Fertility, however, did not differ between groups (77%, 82%, and 74% for C, G1, and G3, respectively; $p = 0.678$).

Milk yield increased from the 1st (32 ± 4 g/d) to the 18th day post-partum (164 ± 4 g/d; $p < 0.001$) in all groups (Figure 4), although, G1 showed the highest marginal means (112 ± 9 g/d, 122 ± 9 g/d, and 111 ± 8 g/d for the C, G1, and G3 groups, respectively; $p < 0.05$).

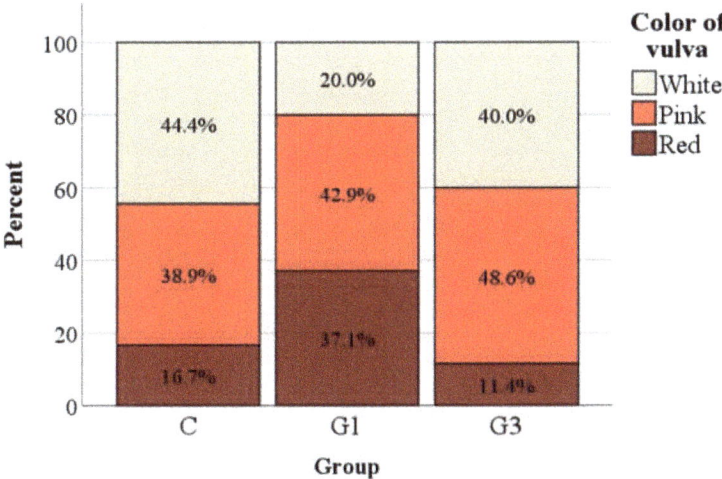

**Figure 3.** Relative frequency distribution of the color of the vulva used as an indicator of sexual receptivity in does of the control group (C) and does supplemented with 1% (G1) or 3% (G3) of Goji.

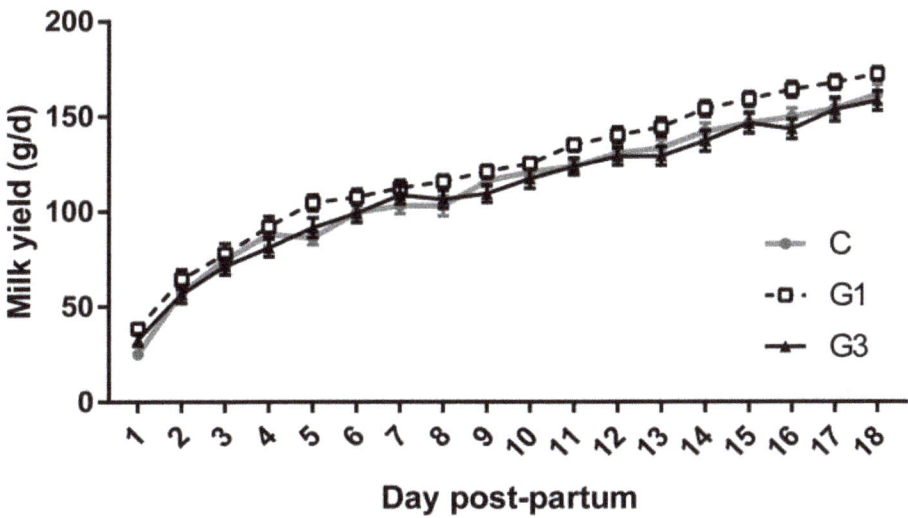

**Figure 4.** Milk production from day 1 to 18 post-partum of the control group (C) and does supplemented with 1% (G1) or 3% (G3) of Goji. Values are means and standard errors.

Pre-weaning mortality ($p = 0.176$) and litter size at birth ($p = 0.249$) did not differ between groups; however, rabbits of the G1 group showed higher litter size at weaning ($p = 0.020$), as well as higher litter weight at birth ($p = 0.008$) and at weaning ($p < 0.001$) compared to the C group. The G3 group showed intermediate values in litter weight at birth and litter size at weaning ($p < 0.05$), while their litter weight at weaning was higher than the C group ($p < 0.01$; Table 2).

Table 2. Productive performance of the control group (C) and does supplemented with 1% (G1) or 3% (G3) of Goji ($n$ = 25 does/group).

| Parameter | C | G1 | G3 | RMSE | $p$ Value |
|---|---|---|---|---|---|
| Pre-weaning mortality (%) | 25.1 | 16.7 | 22.8 | 16.1 | 0.176 |
| Litter size at birth ($n$) | 6.5 | 7.2 | 6.4 | 1.9 | 0.249 |
| Litter weight at birth (g) | 339 [a] | 408 [b] | 356 [ab] | 80 | 0.008 |
| Litter size at weaning ($n$) | 4.8 [a] | 6.0 [b] | 4.9 [ab] | 1.6 | 0.020 |
| Litter weight at weaning (g) | 3634 [a] | 5579 [b] | 4966 [b] | 1255 | <0.001 |

RMSE: root-mean-square error. a: b: Means sharing the same superscript are not significantly different from each other ($p$ < 0.05).

## 4. Discussion

To our knowledge, this is the first study that evaluates the effect of goji berry on the reproductive activity of rabbit does. The present work suggests that the diet integration with goji berry could affect the hormonal pattern of LH and 17β-oestradiol, increase receptivity, milk production, litter weight at birth, litter weight, and size at weaning. The encouraging findings of our research indicate that the berry could be used in rabbit nutrition, although further studies are needed to confirm the current outcomes, in order to understand the mechanism of action as well as to evaluate the economic convenience of its use.

It has long been assumed that rabbit does do not have a well-defined estrus cycle, nor do they show well-specified estrus manifestation, so they are quite often erroneously considered to be in permanent estrus. Actually, the does present a period during which they accept mating (oestrus) as well as a period during which they reject the male (dioestrus). Sexual receptivity could be measured by a behavioral test in the presence of a male [51], and by evaluating the color and turgidity of the vulva [46]. In particular, the mating acceptance behavior in the presence of a male (lordosis position) and the red color of the vulva could be considered as estral manifestations of the doe. The relationships between sexual behavior, vulva color, and circulating concentrations of reproductive hormones have been studied at different reproductive stages, but a firm conclusion has not yet been reached [52,53]. Our results showed that, based on the evaluation of the color of the vulva, the sexual receptivity is higher in supplemented does, namely in the G1 group compared to the C group. Moreover, animals of the same group also showed higher 17β-oestradiol plasma concentrations compared to the other groups at the moment of AI, suggesting a link with the receptivity. In agreement with our findings, the results of several studies highlight that the turgidity and the red color of the vulva, and more in general, the receptive behavior of the doe, can be related to high plasma levels of estradiol [54] as well as to the presence of ovulatory follicles in the ovaries [52]. In fact, the presence of tertiary follicles in the ovaries are responsible for the elevated 17β-oestradiol plasma concentrations, which in turn induce physiological changes in the reproductive organs, such as hyperemia at the vulvar level and act on the hypothalamus which induces the behavioral estrus signals that lead to the acceptance of the male [55]. Moreover, it is quite well-defined that the color of the vulva at the AI greatly influences fertility [56] and ovulation frequency [40]. In our study, although the receptivity and 17β-oestradiol plasma levels showed differences between the groups, they are not correlated with an increase in fertility. The lack of significance for the fertility of the rabbit does, however, could also be affected by the high sensitivity of the chi-square test comparative to the sample size. It was reported that *Lyceum barbarum* polysaccharides were able to restore the production of sex steroids in the ovaries of female senile rats [41]. Moreover, Liu et al. [40] found that *Lycium barbarum* polysaccharide improved the ratio between the different types of follicles, increased the litter size, weaning survival, and hormonal secretion, and reduced the damage of the ovary during repeated superovulation in mice. It was also reported that the administration of an extract of *Lycium chinense Miller* induced ovulation in adult female rabbits [57]. Based on our findings, goji berry seems to be able to enhance sexual receptivity and affects the estrogen secretion of rabbit does. It would also be interesting to evaluate the effect of the supplementation of the fruit on the primiparous and lactating does, in which the receptivity and fertility are usually reduced for their higher negative energy balance and the inhibitory effect of prolactin secretion on the hypothalamus. This preliminary result can encourage the research to explore a possible role of goji berry in the preparation of female rabbits to AI, with the aim to reduce the use of exogenous hormones in rabbit farms. Nonetheless, further investigation is required to confirm these results and to establish the mechanism of action of the goji fruit, given the scarce literature on this topic.

To our knowledge, this is the first report that describes the effect of goji berry on the pattern of LH secretion in rabbits. In the present study, goji berry seems to affect the gonadal axis activity by modifying the LH secretion and the estrogenic activity of the ovary. The rabbit is an induced ovulatory species, in which ovulation is induced by the neuro-endocrine reflex. The penile intromission, mounting, and pheromones induce the release of GnRH in a higher pulse-frequency from the medial basal hypothalamus that acts on the GnRH receptors on the gonadotropic cells in the anterior pituitary and determines the LH ovulatory peak within 15–75 minutes [58,59]. In our study, the exogenous administration of GnRH bypassed the neuro-endocrine ovulatory reflex, acting directly on the gonadotropic cells triggering LH release. In the present study, the LH ovulatory peak occurred within 60 minutes by the injection of synthetic gonadotropin in all the groups. These findings are similar to those reported by Brecchia et al. [49], that also found similar values of LH plasma concentrations after the induction of the ovulation. With respect to our results, other authors showed differences in the LH plasma levels detected and/or on the time of the peak of the gonadotropin after the injection of the GnRH analogs, probably linked to a different method of assay or to an individual variation among the animals [60,61].

In our study, the G1 group tended to differentiate from G3 and C in LH mean concentrations and LH AUC, respectively. The effect of goji berry on the LH concentration has been poorly investigated in humans and animals, in particular in the female. Several studies evaluated the effect of goji berry on the male reproductive tract and hormone concentrations in other species. The administration of goji berry polysaccharides reduced the testis spermatic injury induced by Bisphenol A and significantly increased the LH plasma levels of male mice [62]. Another study showed that *Lycium barbarum* polysaccharides exhibited a protective effect on fertility and reproductive hormone secretion impairments by activating the gonadal axis in streptozotocin-induced type-1 diabetic male mice [63]. Goji berry polysaccharides had protective effects against damage to the testicular tissue, annexed glands, and LH, FSH, and testosterone secretion of normal and hemicastrated male rats induced by heat exposure (43 °C), and on the DNA damage to mouse testicular cells induced by hydrogen peroxide [64]. Recent research showed that dietary integration with goji berry had positive effects on boar semen quality; in particular, it improved progressive motility, total abnormality rate, sperm concentration, and total sperm per ejaculate compared to the control group [65]. Moreover, the wolfberry group showed a significant reduction of the head, tail, and total abnormality rates in both fresh semen and semen stored for 72 hr in comparison to the control group [65]. Finally, it was reported that goji polysaccharides improved sperm quality and fertility rate after cryopreservation in male Cashmere goats [39]. These findings support the idea that goji berry may affect the reproductive hormonal secretion, and as a consequence, the reproductive performance of the animals, including rabbits. It remains to be established which component could be responsible for the action on the gonadal axis of rabbit does as well as the site and the mechanism of action. An up-regulation of the pituitary receptors and/or increased secretion of GnRH secretory neurons, or the synthesis of LH by the gonadotropic cells of the pituitary, might be speculated.

In the present research, we found that a low dose of goji berry integration increases milk production and the weight of the litter at birth and weaning. These results are in agreement and confirm the data reported by Menchetti et al. [47], though they used a smaller sample size. Given the missing data on this topic, we can speculate that some components of the *Lycium barbarum* berry may favor the production of milk in different ways, as reported for other nutraceutical substances in other animal species: increasing the concentration of the components and precursors of milk at the level of the mammary gland [66], stimulating the proliferation of the mammary epithelial cells enhancing the uptake of some precursors of milk such as propionate and butyrate [67], enhancing the secretion of some hormones such as prolactin [68], and acting as key regulators of the signal transduction pathways during the synthesis of the components of milk [69]. Goji berry is rich in free amino acids, particularly in L-arginine [70] which is able to increase milk production in cows [67] and sows [68].

The energy balance of the does in commercial rabbit farms is generally critical. In fact, females are quite often inseminated during lactation when a high energy output is present because of the milk secretion. The loss of energy is not completely compensated for by feed intake, and consequently, the does increase the mobilization of fat reserves and lose energy which negatively affects the reproductive activity [71]. Several metabolic hormones and metabolites are involved in maintaining energy homeostasis during both pregnancy and lactation in rabbit does [26,27]. These hormones and metabolites acting by complex interactions can influence the ovarian axis hormonal secretion, and as a consequence, they play a role in the relationship between energy balance and reproductive efficiency [27]. Moreover, the development of the mammary gland and milk secretion is under hormonal control in adult rabbits [72]. Milk production is influenced mostly by the reproductive (estrogens, progesterone, and prolactin) and metabolic (GH, corticosteroids, thyroid hormones, and insulin) hormones [73]. It was shown that goji berry affects the secretion pattern of metabolic signals such as leptin, insulin, NEFA, and glucose, improving energy homeostasis [22]. Moreover, *Lycium barbarum* has therapeutic effects in glucosides of Tripterygium wilfordii Hook f (GTW)-induced dyszoospermia rats, improving the semen quality and positively affecting the secretion of reproductive hormones, including prolactin [74]. Consequently, it might be suggested that the higher milk yield in the group supplemented with 1% of goji compared to control does in our study can be due to the hormonal framework of both reproductive and metabolic hormone levels.

Our findings showed that the does fed with goji berry had a higher litter size at weaning. Other authors found that a low percentage of goji berry induced lower pre-weaning mortality and, at the same time, higher litter size and weight at the opening of the nest (day 18) and at weaning (day 35) compared to animals fed without goji berry supplement [47]. In the same study, the rabbits that received a diet integrated with goji berry exhibited not only a higher mean body weight during the fattening period and at slaughter, but also a better feed conversion rate compared to control animals. The higher quantity of milk ingested by the litters belonging to the goji groups is probably responsible for the greater productive performance. In fact, a link between the quantity and quality of milk produced by the female and the growth performance of the litter, at least until the weaning was reported [68]. It should be noted that rabbits supplemented with the highest dose of goji berry (i.e., 3%) showed no relevant effects compared to the control group; however, they showed minor changes compared to those obtained with the lowest dose. Then, a non-linear dose-dependent effect was found confirming that the use of high percentages of goji requires further investigation. It has been shown, for example, that substances contained in the *Lycium barbarum*, such as polyphenols, may have negative effects when they reach high levels or are administered for long periods, altering the hormonal and/or energy balance in both male and female farm animals [47,75]. In particular, polyphenols could have estrogen-agonistic or antagonistic effects and could interfere with reproductive functions at different levels of the gonadal axis [75]. However, the effects of polyphenols could be species-specific and depend on the polyphenol profile of each plant [75].

The effects of goji berry dietary supplementation in livestock animals are limited, but there is evidence that the fruit can enhance growth performance in piglets [76], broiler chickens [20], and hybrid groupers [77]. It was reported that some components of the fruit can enhance the intestinal absorption of nutrients [78] and show antioxidant and immunomodulatory actions [79]. There is evidence that *Lycium barbarum* induces changes in the intestinal microbiota, which in turn, can favor the digestion and the absorption of the nutrients [20,80]. Moreover, goji berry polysaccharides can stimulate the gut immune system, increasing the defense of the animals against pathogen infection through direct and indirect actions such as competition for common nutrients and niches and the increase of host defense, respectively [20,75]. Polysaccharides, acting as a prebiotic, favor the growth of beneficial bacteria, which in turn stimulate the immune system and in particular, the innate immune response [81]. It is possible to suggest that the different compounds of goji berry included in the milk and in the feed may stimulate the growth of the animals, influencing the digestion and absorption of the feed by action on the intestinal microbial population. Moreover, the microbiota affecting the development, maturation, and response of the immune system, may contribute to reducing the infectious disease and the mortality of the rabbit. Taken together, these mechanisms can explain the positive effects of goji berry on the growth performance, and more in general, may contribute to the maintenance of good health status and animal welfare.

## 5. Conclusions

In conclusion, the present study provided experimental support for the effects of goji berry on the hormonal profile as well as the reproductive and productive performance of rabbit does. In particular, 1% goji supplementation influences the hormonal pattern and increases both receptivity and milk production of the does, as well as the growth of young rabbits, although the effects on fertility are limited.

Therefore, the use of this natural and nutraceutical product could represent a new strategy to reduce the use of drugs in animal farming. At the same time, it could represent an added value, not only for animal welfare as well as their productive and reproductive performance but also for the rabbit industry and breeding. Although these preliminary findings are encouraging and suggest a potential use of the berries on rabbit nutrition, further studies with a larger number of animals are required to definitely establish both the efficacy and the mechanism of action of the goji berry to improve the reproductive performance of rabbit does, as well as to make a cost-analysis to assess the sustainability of its use in rabbit breeding. In addition, the dose-effect of goji berries could be very interesting for further research.

**Author Contributions:** Conceptualization, E.A., G.C., and G.B.; Data curation, O.B. and E.C.; Formal analysis, L.M., R.Z., and E.C.; Funding acquisition, D.V., M.F., and G.B.; Investigation, S.A., O.B., R.Z., M.R.C., and M.C.; Methodology, E.A., G.C., L.M., and G.B.; Project administration, G.B.; Resources, E.A., D.V., M.F., and G.B.; Software, L.M. and M.F.; Supervision, G.C. and G.B.; Validation, G.B.; Visualization, L.M.; Writing—original draft, G.C., L.M., A.Q., and G.B.; Writing—review and editing, E.A., G.C., L.M., D.V., A.Q., and G.B. All authors have read and agreed to the published version of the manuscript.

**Funding:** This research received no external funding.

**Institutional Review Board Statement:** The experimental protocol was run with the permission of the Ministry of Agriculture and Rural Development, National Authority of Veterinary and Plants protection (prot. 824/2020), of Albania. Every effort has been made to reduce animal discomfort and to use only the number of animals sufficient to produce valid results.

**Informed Consent Statement:** Not applicable.

**Data Availability Statement:** The data presented in this study are available on request from the corresponding author.

**Acknowledgments:** Goji Berries were gently provided by Impresa Agricola of Gianluca Bazzica, Foligno (Italy). The authors acknowledge support from the University of Milan through the APC initiative. The authors wish also to thank Giovanni Migni for his excellent technical assistance.

**Conflicts of Interest:** The authors declare no conflict of interest. The funders had no role in the design of the study; in the collection, analyses, or interpretation of data; in the writing of the manuscript, or in the decision to publish the results.

## References

1. Tian, X.; Liang, T.; Liu, Y.; Ding, G.; Zhang, F.; Ma, Z. Extraction, structural characterization, and biological functions of lycium barbarum polysaccharides: A review. *Biomolecules* **2019**, *9*, 389. [CrossRef]
2. Gao, Y.; Wei, Y.; Wang, Y.; Gao, F.; Chen, Z. Lycium barbarum: A traditional Chinese herb and a promising anti-aging agent. *Aging Dis.* **2017**, *8*, 778–791. [CrossRef]
3. Ma, Z.F.; Zhang, H.; Teh, S.S.; Wang, C.W.; Zhang, Y.; Hayford, F.; Wang, L.; Ma, T.; Dong, Z.; Zhang, Y.; et al. Goji Berries as a potential natural antioxidant medicine: An insight into their molecular mechanisms of action. *Oxid. Med. Cell. Longev.* **2019**, *2019*, 1–9. [CrossRef] [PubMed]
4. Zhao, X.; Guo, S.; Lu, Y.; Hua, Y.; Zhang, F.; Yan, H.; Shang, E.; Wang, H.; Zhang, W.; Duan, J. *Lycium barbarum* L. leaves ameliorate type 2 diabetes in rats by modulating metabolic profiles and gut microbiota composition. *Biomed. Pharmacother.* **2020**, *121*, 109559. [CrossRef]
5. Masci, A.; Carradori, S.; Casadei, M.A.; Paolicelli, P.; Petralito, S.; Ragno, R.; Cesa, S. *Lycium barbarum* polysaccharides: Extraction, purification, structural characterisation and evidence about hypoglycaemic and hypolipidaemic effects. A review. *Food Chem.* **2018**, *254*, 377–389. [CrossRef]
6. Ceccarini, M.R.; Vannini, S.; Cataldi, S.; Moretti, M.; Villarini, M.; Fioretti, B.; Albi, E.; Beccari, T.; Codini, M. Effect of *Lycium barbarum* berries cultivated in Umbria (Italy) on human hepatocellular carcinoma cells. *J. Biotechnol.* **2016**, *231*, S26–S27. [CrossRef]
7. Yu, M.S.; Ho, Y.S.; So, K.F.; Yuen, W.H.; Chang, R.C.C. Cytoprotective effects of *Lycium barbarum* against reducing stress on endoplasmic reticulum. *Int. J. Mol. Med.* **2006**, *17*, 1157–1161. [CrossRef] [PubMed]
8. Xing, X.; Liu, F.; Xiao, J.; So, K.F. Neuro-protective Mechanisms of *Lycium barbarum*. *NeuroMolecular Med.* **2016**, *18*, 253–263. [CrossRef]
9. Ceccarini, M.R.; Codini, M.; Cataldi, S.; Vannini, S.; Lazzarini, A.; Floridi, A.; Moretti, M.; Villarini, M.; Fioretti, B.; Beccari, T.; et al. Acid sphingomyelinase as target of Lycium Chinense: Promising new action for cell health. *Lipids Health Dis.* **2016**, *15*, 183. [CrossRef]
10. Bo, R.; Sun, Y.; Zhou, S.; Ou, N.; Gu, P.; Liu, Z.; Hu, Y.; Liu, J.; Wang, D. Simple nanoliposomes encapsulating *Lycium barbarum* polysaccharides as adjuvants improve humoral and cellular immunity in mice. *Int. J. Nanomedicine* **2017**, *12*, 6289–6301. [CrossRef]
11. Lian, Y.Z.; Lin, I.H.; Yang, Y.C.; Chao, J.C.J. Gastroprotective effect of *Lycium barbarum* polysaccharides and C-phyocyanin in rats with ethanol-induced gastric ulcer. *Int. J. Biol. Macromol.* **2020**, *165*, 1519–1528. [CrossRef]
12. Reeve, V.E.; Allanson, M.; Arun, S.J.; Domanski, D.; Painter, N. Mice drinking goji berry juice (*Lycium barbarum*) are protected from UV radiation-induced skin damage via antioxidant pathways. *Photochem. Photobiol. Sci.* **2010**, *9*, 601–607. [CrossRef]
13. Liu, L.; Sha, X.Y.; Wu, Y.N.; Chen, M.T.; Zhong, J.X. *Lycium barbarum* polysaccharides protects retinal ganglion cells against oxidative stress injury. *Neural Regen. Res.* **2020**, *15*, 1526–1531. [CrossRef]
14. Amagase, H.; Farnsworth, N.R. A review of botanical characteristics, phytochemistry, clinical relevance in efficacy and safety of *Lycium barbarum* fruit (Goji). *Food Res. Int.* **2011**, *44*, 1702–1717. [CrossRef]
15. Kwok, S.S.; Bu, Y.; Lo, A.C.Y.; Chan, T.C.Y.; So, K.F.; Lai, J.S.M.; Shih, K.C. A Systematic Review of Potential Therapeutic Use of Lycium Barbarum Polysaccharides in Disease. *Biomed Res. Int.* **2019**, *4615745*. [CrossRef]
16. Carnés, J.; De Larramendi, C.H.; Ferrer, A.; Huertas, A.J.; López-Matas, M.A.; Pagán, J.A.; Navarro, L.A.; García-Abujeta, J.L.; Vicario, S.; Peña, M. Recently introduced foods as new allergenic sources: Sensitisation to Goji berries (Lycium barbarum). *Food Chem.* **2013**, *137*, 130–135. [CrossRef] [PubMed]
17. Endes, Z.; Uslu, N.; Özcan, M.M.; Er, F. Physico-chemical properties, fatty acid composition and mineral contents of goji berry (*Lycium barbarum* L.) fruit. *J. Agroaliment. Process. Technol.* **2015**, *21*, 36–40.
18. Wang, C.C.; Chang, S.C.; Inbaraj, B.S.; Chen, B.H. Isolation of carotenoids, flavonoids and polysaccharides from *Lycium barbarum* L. and evaluation of antioxidant activity. *Food Chem.* **2010**, *120*, 184–192. [CrossRef]
19. Filipescu, I.E.; Leonardi, L.; Menchetti, L.; Guelfi, G.; Traina, G.; Casagrande-Proietti, P.; Piro, F.; Quattrone, A.; Barbato, O.; Brecchia, G. Preventive effects of bovine colostrum supplementation in TNBS-induced colitis in mice. *PLoS ONE* **2018**, *13*, 1–17. [CrossRef] [PubMed]
20. Long, L.N.; Kang, B.J.; Jiang, Q.; Chen, J.S. Effects of dietary Lycium barbarum polysaccharides on growth performance, digestive enzyme activities, antioxidant status, and immunity of broiler chickens. *Poult. Sci.* **2020**, *99*, 744–751. [CrossRef]
21. Menchetti, L.; Brecchia, G.; Branciari, R.; Barbato, O.; Fioretti, B.; Codini, M.; Bellezza, E.; Trabalza-Marinucci, M.; Miraglia, D. The effect of Goji berries (Lycium barbarum) dietary supplementation on rabbit meat quality. *Meat. Sci.* **2020**, *161*, 108018. [CrossRef]
22. Menchetti, L.; Curone, G.; Andoni, E.; Barbato, O.; Troisi, A.; Fioretti, B.; Polisca, A.; Codini, M.; Canali, C.; Vigo, D.; et al. Impact of goji berries (*Lycium barbarum*) supplementation on the energy homeostasis of rabbit does: Uni- and multivariate approach. *Animals* **2020**, *10*, 2000. [CrossRef]
23. Castrica, M.; Menchetti, L.; Balzaretti, C.C.M.; Branciari, R.; Ranucci, D.; Cotozzolo, E.; Vigo, D.; Curone, G.; Brecchia, G.; Miraglia, D. Impact of dietary supplementation with goji berries (Lycium barbarum) on microbiological quality, physico-chemical, and sensory characteristics of rabbit meat. *Foods* **2020**, *9*, 1480. [CrossRef] [PubMed]

24. Rommers, J.M.; Boiti, C.; Brecchia, G.; Meijerhof, R.; Noordhuizen, J.P.T.M.; Decuypere, E.; Kemp, B. Metabolic adaptation and hormonal regulation in young rabbit does during long-term caloric restriction and subsequent compensatory growth. *Anim. Sci.* **2004**, *79*, 255–264. [CrossRef]
25. Martínez-Paredes, E.; Ródenas, L.; Martínez-Vallespín, B.; Cervera, C.; Blas, E.; Brecchia, G.; Boiti, C.; Pascual, J.J. Effects of feeding programme on the performance and energy balance of nulliparous rabbit does. *Animal* **2012**, *6*, 1086–1095. [CrossRef] [PubMed]
26. Menchetti, L.; Brecchia, G.; Canali, C.; Cardinali, R.; Polisca, A.; Zerani, M.; Boiti, C. Food restriction during pregnancy in rabbits: Effects on hormones and metabolites involved in energy homeostasis and metabolic programming. *Res. Vet. Sci.* **2015**, *98*, 7–12. [CrossRef]
27. Menchetti, L.; Andoni, E.; Barbato, O.; Canali, C.; Quattrone, A.; Vigo, D.; Codini, M.; Curone, G.; Brecchia, G. Energy homeostasis in rabbit does during pregnancy and pseudopregnancy. *Anim. Reprod. Sci.* **2020**, *218*, 106505. [CrossRef]
28. Menchetti, L.; Barbato, O.; Filipescu, I.E.; Traina, G.; Leonardi, L.; Polisca, A.; Troisi, A.; Guelfi, G.; Piro, F.; Brecchia, G. Effects of local lipopolysaccharide administration on the expression of Toll-like receptor 4 and pro-inflammatory cytokines in uterus and oviduct of rabbit does. *Theriogenology* **2018**, *107*, 162–174. [CrossRef] [PubMed]
29. Boiti, C.; Canali, C.; Brecchia, G.; Zanon, F.; Facchin, E. Effects of induced endometritis on the life-span of corpora lutea in pseudopregnant rabbits and incidence of spontaneous uterine infections related to fertility of breeding does. *Theriogenology* **1999**, *52*, 1123–1132. [CrossRef]
30. Cronin, J.G.; Turner, M.L.; Goetze, L.; Bryant, C.E.; Sheldon, I.M. Toll-Like Receptor 4 and MYD88-Dependent Signaling Mechanisms of the Innate Immune System Are Essential for the Response to Lipopolysaccharide by Epithelial and Stromal Cells of the Bovine Endometrium1. *Biol. Reprod.* **2012**, *86*, 51. [CrossRef] [PubMed]
31. Brecchia, G.; Menchetti, L.; Cardinali, R.; Castellini, C.; Polisca, a.; Zerani, M.; Maranesi, M.; Boiti, C. Effects of a bacterial lipopolysaccharide on the reproductive functions of rabbit does. *Anim. Reprod. Sci.* **2014**, *147*, 128–134. [CrossRef] [PubMed]
32. Brecchia, G.; Cardinali, R.; Mourvaki, E.; Collodel, G.; Moretti, E.; Dal Bosco, A.; Castellini, C. Short- and long-term effects of lipopolysaccharide-induced inflammation on rabbit sperm quality. *Anim. Reprod. Sci.* **2010**, *118*, 310–316. [CrossRef]
33. Roth, N.; Käsbohrer, A.; Mayrhofer, S.; Zitz, U.; Hofacre, C.; Domig, K.J. The application of antibiotics in broiler production and the resulting antibiotic resistance in Escherichia coli: A global overview. *Poult. Sci.* **2019**, *98*, 1791–1804. [CrossRef] [PubMed]
34. Oliver, J.P.; Gooch, C.A.; Lansing, S.; Schueler, J.; Hurst, J.J.; Sassoubre, L.; Crossette, E.M.; Aga, D.S. Invited review: Fate of antibiotic residues, antibiotic-resistant bacteria, and antibiotic resistance genes in US dairy manure management systems. *J. Dairy Sci.* **2020**, *103*, 1051–1071. [CrossRef]
35. Amore, G.; Beloeil, P.; Bocca, V.; Boelaert, F.; Gibin, D.; Papanikolaou, A.; Rizz, V.; Stoicescu, A. Zoonoses, antimicrobial resistance and food-borne outbreaks guidance for reporting 2020 data. *EFSA Support. Publ.* **2021**, *18*, 112. [CrossRef]
36. Menchetti, L.; Barbato, O.; Sforna, M.; Vigo, D.; Mattioli, S.; Curone, G.; Tecilla, M.; Riva, F.; Brecchia, G. Effects of Diets Enriched in Linseed and Fish Oil on the Expression Pattern of Toll-Like Receptors 4 and Proinflammatory Cytokines on Gonadal Axis and Reproductive Organs in Rabbit Buck. *Oxid. Med. Cell. Longev.* **2020**, *2020*, 4327470. [CrossRef] [PubMed]
37. Freitas, M.L.; De Oliveira, R.A. Nutraceutical in male reproduction. *Rev. Bras. Med. Vet.* **2018**, *40*, e220118. [CrossRef]
38. Liu, C.; Gu, J.; Ma, W.; Zhang, Q.; Song, M.; Ha, L.; Xu, X.; Jiao, H.; Huo, Z. Lycium barbarum polysaccharide protects against ethanol-induced spermiotoxicity and testicular degenera-tion in Immp2l(+/-) mice. *Andrologia* **2020**, *52*, e13554. [CrossRef]
39. Ren, F.; Fang, Q.; Feng, T.; Li, Y.; Wang, Y.; Zhu, H.; Hu, J. *Lycium barbarum* and *Laminaria japonica* polysaccharides improve Cashmere goat sperm quality and fertility rate after cryopreservation. *Theriogenology* **2019**, *129*, 29–36. [CrossRef]
40. Liu, B.; Wang, J.L.; Wang, X.M.; Zhang, C.; Dai, J.G.; Huang, X.M.; Gao, J.M. Reparative effects of lycium barbarum polysaccharide on mouse ovarian injuries induced by repeated superovulation. *Theriogenology* **2020**, *145*, 115–125. [CrossRef]
41. Wei, M.; ZHeng, S.; Ma, H.; Lv, Y. Discussion of protective mechanism of Lyceum barbarum polysaccharides on ovarian tissue in female senile rats. *Zhong Yao Cai* **2011**, *34*, 1915–1918.
42. Polisca, A.; Scotti, L.; Orlandi, R.; Brecchia, G.; Boiti, C. Doppler evaluation of maternal and fetal vessels during normal gestation in rabbits. *Theriogenology* **2010**, *73*, 358–366. [CrossRef] [PubMed]
43. Boiti, C.; Guelfi, G.; Zerani, M.; Zampini, D.; Brecchia, G.; Gobbetti, A. Expression patterns of cytokines, p53 and nitric oxide synthase isoenzymes in corpora lutea of pseudopregnant rabbits during spontaneous luteolysis. *Reproduction* **2004**, *127*, 229–238. [CrossRef]
44. Parillo, F.; Dall'Aglio, C.; Brecchia, G.; Maranesi, M.; Polisca, A.; Boiti, C.; Zerani, M. Aglepristone (RU534) effects on luteal function of pseudopregnant rabbits: Steroid receptors, enzymatic activities, and hormone productions in corpus luteum and uterus. *Anim. Reprod. Sci.* **2013**, *138*, 118–132. [CrossRef] [PubMed]
45. Maertens, L.; Moermans, R.; De Groote, G. Prediction of the apparent digestible energy content of commercial pelleted feeds for rabbits. *J. Appl. Rabbit. Res.* **1988**, *11*, 60–67.
46. IRRG; Theau-Clément, M.; Maertens, L.; Castellini, C.; Besenfelder, U.; Boiti, C. Recommendations and guidelines for applied reproduction trials with rabbit does. *World Rabbit Sci.* **2005**, *13*, 147–164.
47. Menchetti, L.; Vecchione, L.; Filipescu, I.; Petrescu, V.F.; Fioretti, B.; Beccari, T.; Ceccarini, M.R.; Codini, M.; Quattrone, A.; Trabalza-Marinucci, M.; et al. Effects of Goji berries supplementation on the productive performance of rabbit. *Livest. Sci.* **2019**, *220*, 123–128. [CrossRef]

48. Menchetti, L.; Canali, C.; Castellini, C.; Boiti, C.; Brecchia, G. The different effects of linseed and fish oil supplemented diets on insulin sensitivity of rabbit does during pregnancy. *Res. Vet. Sci.* **2018**, *118*, 126–133. [CrossRef]
49. Brecchia, G.; Bonanno, A.; Galeati, G.; Federici, C.; Maranesi, M.; Gobbetti, A.; Zerani, M.; Boiti, C. Hormonal and metabolic adaptation to fasting: Effects on the hypothalamic-pituitary-ovarian axis and reproductive performance of rabbit does. *Domest. Anim. Endocrinol.* **2006**, *31*, 105–122. [CrossRef]
50. Troisi, A.; Polisca, A.; Cardinali, L.; Orlandi, R.; Brecchia, G.; Menchetti, L.; Zerani, M.; Maranesi, M.; Di Mari, W.; Verstegen, J.P. Effect of aglepristone (RU534) administration during follicular phase on progesterone, estradiol-17β and LH serum concentrations in bitches. *Reprod. Domest. Anim.* **2020**, *55*, 1794–1802. [CrossRef]
51. Moret, B. Comportement d'oestrus chez la lapine. *Cunicult. Mag.* **1980**, *33*, 159–161.
52. Rodriguez, J.M.; Ubilla, E. Effects of sexual receptivity on ovulation response in rabbit does induced with GnRH. In Proceedings of the Proc 4th World Rabbit Congress, Buadapest, Hungary, 10–14 October 1988; pp. 504–509.
53. Stouflet, I.; Caillol, M. Relation between circulating sex steroid concentrations and sexual behaviour during pregnancy and post-partum in the domestic rabbit. *J. Reprod. Fertil.* **1988**, *82*, 209–218. [CrossRef]
54. Rebollar, P.G.; Ubilla, E.; Alvarino, J.M.R.; Illera, J.C.; Silvan, G. Effect of degree of sexual receptivity on post-partum plasma estardiol and ovulatory response in rabbit. *Rev. Esp. Fisiol.* **1992**, *43*, 13–18.
55. Caillol, M.; Dauphin-Villemant, C.; Martinet, L. Oestrous behaviour and circulating progesterone and oestrogen levels during pseudo-pregnancy in the domestic rabbit. *J. Reprod. Fertil.* **1983**, *69*, 179–186. [CrossRef] [PubMed]
56. Roustan, M.A. A study on relationship between receptivity and lactation in the doe, and their influ-ence on reproductive performance. *J. Appl. Rabbit. Res.* **1992**, *15*, 412–421.
57. Suzuki, M.; Osawa, S.; Hirano, M. A Lycium Chinense Miller Component Inducing Ovulation in Adult Female Rabbits. *Tohoku J. Exp. Med.* **1972**, *106*, 219–231. [CrossRef]
58. Pau, K.; Orstead, K.; Hess, D.; Spies, H. Feedback effects of ovarian steroids on the hypothalamic-hypophyseal axis in the rab-bit. *Biol. Reprod.* **1986**, *35*, 1009–1023. [CrossRef] [PubMed]
59. Ramirez, V.; Soufi, W. The neuroendocrine control of the rabbit ovarian cycle. In *The Physiology of Reproduction*, 2nd ed.; Knobil, E., Neill, J.D., Eds.; Raven Press: New York, NY, US, 1994; pp. 585–611.
60. Rebollar, P.; Dal Bosco, A.; Millán, P.; Cardinali, R.; Brecchia, G.; Sylla, L.; Lorenzo, P.; Castellini, C. Ovulating induction methods in rabbit does: The pituitary and ovarian responses. *Theriogenology* **2012**, *77*, 292–298. [CrossRef]
61. Jones, E.E.; Bain, J.B.; Odell, W.D. Postcoital luteinizing hormone release in male and female rabbits as determined by ra-dioimmunoassay. *Fertil. Steril.* **1976**, 848–852. [CrossRef]
62. Zhang, C.; Wang, A.; Sun, X.; Li, X.; Zhao, X.; Li, S.; Ma, A. Protective effects of lycium barbarum polysaccharides on testis spermatogenic injury induced by bisphenol a in mice. *Evidence Based Complement. Altern. Med.* **2013**, *2013*, 690808. [CrossRef]
63. Shi, G.J.; Zheng, J.; Wu, J.; Qiao, H.Q.; Chang, Q.; Niu, Y.; Sun, T.; Li, Y.X.; Yu, J.Q. Protective effects of lycium barbarum polysaccharide on male sexual dysfunction and fertility impairments by activating hypothalamic pituitary gonadal axis in streptozotocin-induced type-1 diabetic male mice. *Endocr. J.* **2017**, *64*, 907–922. [CrossRef] [PubMed]
64. Luo, Q.; Li, Z.; Huang, X.; Yan, J.; Zhang, S.; Cai, Y.Z. Lycium barbarum polysaccharides: Protective effects against heat-induced damage of rat testes and H2O2-induced DNA damage in mouse testicular cells and beneficial effect on sexual behavior and reproductive function of hemicastrated rats. *Life Sci.* **2006**, *79*, 613–621. [CrossRef]
65. Yang, Q.; Xing, Y.; Qiao, C.; Liu, W.; Jiang, H.; Fu, Q.; Zhou, Y.; Yang, B.; Zhang, Z.; Chen, R. Semen quality improvement in boars fed with supplemental wolfberry (Lycium barbarum). *Anim. Sci. J.* **2019**, *90*, 1517–1522. [CrossRef] [PubMed]
66. Bauman, D.E.; Mather, I.H.; Wall, R.J.; Lock, A.L. Major advances associated with the biosynthesis of milk. *J. Dairy Sci.* **2006**, *89*, 1235–1243. [CrossRef]
67. Zhang, X.; Wang, Y.; Wang, M.; Zhou, G.; Chen, L.; Ding, L.; Bu, D.; Loor, J. Arginine supply impacts the expression of candidate microRNA controlling milk casein yield in Bovine mammary tissue. *Animals* **2020**, *10*, 797. [CrossRef] [PubMed]
68. Zhu, C.; Guo, C.y.; Gao, K.g.; Wang, L.; Chen, Z.; Ma, X.y.; Jiang, Z.y. Dietary arginine supplementation in multiparous sows during lactation improves the weight gain of suckling piglets. *J. Integr. Agric.* **2017**, *16*, 648–655. [CrossRef]
69. Moshel, Y.; Rhoads, R.E.; Barash, I. Role of amino acids in translational mechanisms governing milk protein synthesis in murine and ruminant mammary epithelial cells. *J. Cell. Biochem.* **2006**, *98*, 685–700. [CrossRef] [PubMed]
70. Potterat, O. Goji (Lycium barbarum and L. chinense): Phytochemistry, pharmacology and safety in the perspective of traditional uses and recent popularity. *Planta Med.* **2010**, *76*, 7–19. [CrossRef]
71. Xiccato, G.; Bernardini, M.; Castellini, C.; Dalle Zotte, A.; Queaque, P.I.; Trocino, A. Effect of postweaning feeding on the performance and energy balance of female rabbits at different physiological states. *J. Anim. Sci.* **1999**, *77*, 416–426. [CrossRef] [PubMed]
72. Svennersten-Sjaunja, K.; Olsson, K. Endocrinology of milk production. *Domest. Anim. Endocrinol.* **2005**, *29*, 241–258. [CrossRef]
73. Szendrö, Z.; Matics, Z.; Brecchia, G.; Theau-Clément, M.; Nagy, Z.; Princz, Z.; Biró-Németh, E.; Radnai, I.; Nagy, I. Milk production of pseudopregnant multiparous does. *World Rabbit Sci.* **2010**, *18*, 77–82. [CrossRef]
74. Guan, S.; Zhu, Y.; Wang, J.; Dong, L.; Zhao, Q.; Wang, L.; Wang, B.; Li, H. A combination of Semen Cuscutae and Fructus Lycii improves testicular cell proliferation and inhibits their apoptosis in rats with spermatogenic dysfunction by regulating the SCF/c-kit–PI3K–Bcl-2 pathway. *J. Ethnopharmacol.* **2020**, *251*, 112525. [CrossRef] [PubMed]

75. Hashem, N.M.; Gonzalez-Bulnes, A.; Simal-Gandara, J. Polyphenols in farm animals: Source of reproductive gain or waste? *Antioxidants* **2020**, *9*, 1023. [CrossRef] [PubMed]
76. Chen, J.; Long, L.; Jiang, Q.; Kang, B.; Li, Y.; Yin, J. Effects of dietary supplementation of Lycium barbarum polysaccharides on growth performance, immune status, antioxidant capacity and selected microbial populations of weaned piglets. *J. Anim. Physiol. Anim. Nutr.* **2020**, *104*, 1106–1115. [CrossRef] [PubMed]
77. Tan, X.; Sun, Z.; Ye, C.; Lin, H. The effects of dietary Lycium barbarum extract on growth performance, liver health and immune related genes expression in hybrid grouper (Epinephelus lanceolatus♂ × E. fuscoguttatus♀) fed high lipid diets. *Fish Shellfish Immunol.* **2019**, *87*, 847–852. [CrossRef]
78. Ren, L.; Li, J.; Xiao, Y.; Zhang, Y.; Fan, J.; Zhang, B.; Wang, L.; Shen, X. Polysaccharide from *Lycium barbarum* L. leaves enhances absorption of endogenous calcium, and elevates cecal calcium transport protein levels and serum cytokine levels in rats. *J. Funct. Foods* **2017**, *33*, 227–234. [CrossRef]
79. Zhu, W.; Zhou, S.; Liu, J.; McLean, R.J.C.; Chu, W. Prebiotic, immuno-stimulating and gut microbiota-modulating effects of Lycium barbarum polysaccharide. *Biomed. Pharmacother.* **2020**, *121*, 109591. [CrossRef]
80. Wang, M.; Xie, Z.; Li, L.; Chen, Y.; Li, Y.; Wang, Y.; Lu, B.; Zhang, S.; Ma, F.; Ma, C.W.; et al. Supplementation with compound polysaccharides contributes to the development and metabolic activity of young rat intestinal microbiota. *Food Funct.* **2019**, *10*, 2658–2675. [CrossRef]
81. Tang, C.; Ding, R.; Sun, J.; Liu, J.; Kan, J.; Jin, C. The impacts of natural polysaccharides on intestinal microbiota and immune responses-a review. *Food Funct.* **2019**, *10*, 2290–2312. [CrossRef]

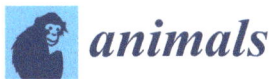

*Review*

# Current Knowledge on the Bioavailability of Thymol as a Feed Additive in Humans and Animals with a Focus on Rabbit Metabolic Processes

Iveta Placha [1,*], Kristina Bacova [1,2] and Lukas Plachy [3,4]

[1] Centre of Biosciences of the Slovak Academy of Sciences, Institute of Animal Physiology, Soltesovej 4-6, 040 01 Kosice, Slovakia; bacovak@saske.sk
[2] University of Veterinary Medicine and Pharmacy, Komenskeho 73, 041 81 Kosice, Slovakia
[3] 1st Department of Cardiology, East Slovak Institute of Cardiovascular Diseases, Ondavska 8, 040 11 Kosice, Slovakia; lukas.plachy@upjs.sk
[4] Faculty of Medicine, Pavol Jozef Safarik University in Kosice, Trieda SNP 457/1, 040 11 Kosice, Slovakia
* Correspondence: placha@saske.sk; Tel.: +421-55-792-2969

**Simple Summary:** This review provides general information on the possible health benefits in animals and humans of herbal additives, particularly thymol, whose phenolic group is responsible for the neutralisation of free radicals, and information concerning its detection through body action, bioavailability and mechanisms in rabbits. Plants containing thymol have been used in traditional medicine for the treatment of various diseases, such as cardiovascular diseases, cancer and diabetes. Although a great number of in vitro studies of cardiovascular and cancer diseases are available, in vivo studies that confirm these findings have not been sufficiently reported. To determine the beneficial dose, further clinical studies are necessary, with preclinical comprehensive research on animal models.

**Abstract:** The aim of this review is to describe the therapeutic effect of thymol on various human diseases, followed by its bioavailability in humans and animals. Based on our knowledge from the current literature, after thymol addition, thymol metabolites—mostly thymol sulphate and glucuronide—are detected in the plasma and urine of humans and in the plasma, intestinal content, faeces and tissues in rats, pigs, chickens, horses and rabbits after enzymatic cleavage. In rabbits, thymol absorption from the gastrointestinal tract, its distribution within the organism, its accumulation in tissues and its excretion from the organism have been described in detail. It is necessary and important for these studies to suggest the appropriate dose needed to achieve the required health benefits not only for animals but also for humans. Information from this review concerning the mode of action of thymol in animal organisms could also be applied to human medicine and may help in the utilisation of herbal medicine in humans and in veterinary healthcare. This review summarises the important aspects of thymol's effects on health and its bioavailability in organisms, particularly in rabbits. In future, herbal-based drugs must be extensively investigated in terms of their mode of action, efficiency of administration and clinical effect.

**Keywords:** thymol; biological activity; health; human; animal

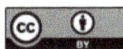

## 1. Introduction

For many years now, the positive effects of aromatic plants and herbs in the treatment of various diseases have been well documented. Many effective and conventional drugs originate from plants, and, historically, they represent the first pharmacological compounds used in the treatment of many diseases [1–3]. Scientists have focused their attention on the composition of herbal extracts, the detection of their active compounds and their mode of action to ensure an effective therapeutic and nutritional dosage [4]. To understand the mechanism of action of these compounds and to determine their interaction with food and drugs, their absorption, distribution, metabolism and excretion all need to be investigated [5,6].

Currently, the widespread antibiotic resistance presents a global health problem, and it has forced medical researchers to return to the pre-antibiotic era [7,8]. For this reason, the development of new drugs of natural origin presents a big challenge for scientists [9,10]. More than half of the drugs approved by Food and Drug Administration (FDA) are composed of natural compounds from medicinal plants [11]. About 50% of modern drugs, and more than 60% of anti-cancer drugs, are developed from phytochemicals [12]. According to Chen et al. [13] and Newman et al. [14], plants and their natural compounds have been used as sources of antibiotics, analgesics, cardioprotective and other drugs for more than 5000 years. Currently, collaboration between the World Health Organization (WHO), the FDA, the European Medicines Agency (EMA) and the pharmaceutical industry is necessary in order to utilise the vast potential of traditional medicine for the development of herbal drugs for the treatment of different diseases [15]. Despite the fact that aromatic plants and herbs are considered natural and safer than synthetic drugs, they may present a risk of serious adverse effects [16]. For this reason, researchers have suggested that food and drug interactions must be extensively evaluated in terms of their absorption, excretion, distribution and metabolism [5,6].

Many gastrointestinal and respiratory diseases in pigs, poultry and young cattle [17–19] and mastitis in adult cattle [20] are very often treated with antibiotics [21]. Bacteria that are spread into the environment by the excrement of farm animals carry antimicrobial resistance genes [22], and they are directly, or by food consumption, transmitted to humans [23,24]. The preventive use of medicinal plants may help to lower the use of antibiotics for the treatment of farm animals [25]. However, this statement is not mentioned in any national strategy on antibiotic resistance [26]. In recent decades, veterinarians and farmers have shown increased interest in using herbal medicine with the goal of reducing the use of antibiotics [27]. In order to explore strategies to minimise the development of antimicrobial resistance, more clinical veterinary studies using medicinal plants are required [21].

In recent years, plant secondary metabolites and plant-derived extracts have received extensive attention. Thymol, a major compound of thyme (*Thymus vulgaris* L.), exhibits antioxidant properties related to its phenolic structure, which adsorbs and neutralises free radicals. Several preclinical studies have well documented the pharmacological properties of thymol on animal models, but thymol also exhibits multi-pharmacological properties against various human diseases [28–31].

Thymol has been evaluated in many studies, which confirmed its therapeutic uses for the treatment of disorders affecting the cardiovascular, nervous, respiratory and digestive systems [32–35].

WHO reported, that cardiovascular diseases accounted for the highest number of deaths in 2019, and they are expected to reach 22.2 million deaths in 2030 [36]. For this reason, finding safe, non-toxic and effective drugs for prevention of these diseases is a hot topic of research. As natural candidates, some medicinal plants could meet the requirements for such pharmacological effects [37]. The active components of medicinal plants, due to their chemical structure and ability to reduce and scavenge the production of free radicals, improve the activity of antioxidant enzymes and are able to downregulate the oxidative stress of the organism [38]. In the opinion of Chang et al. [37], natural medicinal plants could be less toxic than synthetic antioxidants. Accumulating evidence suggests that flavonoids, phenolics and saponin from medical plants could reduce oxidative stress [16]. Moreover, some phenolic phytochemicals have anti-carcinogenic and anti-inflammatory effects [37,39]. Local inflammation and oxidative stress are involved in the pathogenesis of endothelial dysfunction and, consequently, in the progression of atherosclerosis [30]. Oxidative stress, by way of regulating inflammation and stimulating vascular smooth muscle, plays a key role in the pathogenesis of hypertension, atherosclerosis and myocardial injury [37,40–42]. Oxidative stress represents an imbalance between free radical formation and antioxidant defence. An excessive amount of free radicals attack lipids in cells and cause their dysfunction, which induces the process of atherogenesis [43].

De Brito Alves et al. [44] suppose that the dietary intake of phenolic compounds could prevent hypertension through the beneficial impact on the gut microbiome. As much as 90–95% of phenolic compounds are accumulated in the large intestine, where they are converted into active metabolites by gut microbiota and, in turn, can modulate gut microbial composition by supporting the growth of certain beneficial bacteria [45,46]. Natarajan et al. [47] suggested that short-chain fatty acids, the major final product of faecal bacterial activity, could be responsible for lowering blood pressure. However, future studies are necessary to find a relationship between plant-derived phenolic compounds and the gut microbiome in connection with the prevention of hypertension [44,48]. In order to test the possible mechanism of action of these compounds, it would be interesting to design in vitro culture models that simulate intestinal tract conditions or to find a suitable animal model [30,49]. Yu et al. [30] showed that rabbits, in comparison with other laboratory animals, are the most suitable model for the study of atherosclerosis in humans due to their similar lipoprotein metabolism.

The strong antimicrobial properties of thymol have been suggested by several studies. Thymol can be useful in the therapy of intestinal problems and respiratory infections [50]. Based on the studies of Komaki et al. [51] and Asadbegi et al. [52], the extract of *T. vulgaris* is considered as neuroprotective and is used to prevent anxiety. Thymol's phenolic structure neutralises free radicals and exhibits redox properties [30]. In addition to in vitro and in vivo studies, clinical studies are required to establish the most effective way and dosage regimen of thymol administration [50].

To find the therapeutically relevant effects of plant compounds, reliable pharmacokinetic studies in humans are necessary [53]. An appropriate dose that would ensure the expected effect, absorption and excretion of phenolic compounds after thyme extract intake was studied in humans by Rubió et al. [54] and Kohlert et al. [55]. These data may also be important in the context of the safe application of herbal medicinal products [53]. However, relatively few studies on the bioavailability and pharmacokinetics of thymol, particularly in humans, are available to date [55]. To monitor phenolic consumption, hydroxytyrosol metabolites were analysed as a biomarker. However, the results showed its low specificity [54]. The authors showed that the metabolites of thymol, thymol sulphate and glucuronide were more specific, and they established the relationship between exposure and effect more precisely.

Present studies do not only focus their attention on the chemical composition and pharmacology of medicinal plants; their main objectives are the study of metabolites, the products of cell metabolism and their mechanism of action [56]. In order to propose the optimal dosage regimen, it is necessary to take into account that the metabolites of plant compounds could probably be deconjugated to the parental compounds and express their pharmacological activity in this way [54,55]. Thymol sulphate and thymol glucuronide are the main metabolites of thymol, but, unfortunately, there is no information whether these compounds are active or inactive forms [50]. Thyme has often been used in folk medicine, and, recently, scientists have focused their attention on the pharmacodynamic activities of compounds in vitro, as well as their bioavailability in target organs [55].

The present review focuses in greater detail on the application of thymol as a natural feed additive in humans and animals to improve their health, with the aim being to substitute synthetic drugs. The limited information available on the bioactivity of thymol and its metabolites in organisms suggested to us to summarise the current knowledge of its absorption, distribution, accumulation and excretion. In the following sections, we try to compile all of the available literature in order to provide information concerning the tissues in which thymol and its metabolites have been detected to date and to describe the processes of its biotransformation, absorption, distribution, deposition and elimination and bioavailability in human and animal organisms.

## 2. Detection of Thymol and Its Metabolites in Humans and Animals

The pharmacodynamic activities of thyme extract or essential oil have been demonstrated in vitro. To confirm the beneficial effect of thymol found in vitro, its absorption, distribution, metabolism and excretion need to be detected in vivo [55]. To the best of our knowledge, thymol distribution in tissues in vivo has only been detected in more recent studies by several authors. To better understand the bioavailability of thymol in animal organisms and to establish the suitable concentration for beneficial effects on animal health, its metabolic path needs to be understood at the molecular level [57,58]. Little is known about the bioactivity of thymol and its metabolites, as there are only few studies that have analysed thymol in body tissues (Table 1).

According to our knowledge, the first study dealing with the metabolic fate of thymol, particularly its metabolite thymol glucuronide in the urine of rabbits and humans, was studied by Takada et al. [59]. The next early study was the examination of the glucuronide and sulphate conjugates of thymol as well as its isomer carvacrol in rat urine by Austgulen et al. [60]. Kraus and Ternes [61] detected thymol in egg yolk but not in albumin after the addition of thyme extract to laying hens. The transition of thymol from food into the yolk represented 0.006%.

The bioavailability of thymol as the main compound of thyme essential oil after the oral administration of a single dose of Bronchipret® tablets (equivalent to 1.08 mg thymol) to humans was examined by Kohlert et al. [53]. No thymol was detected in plasma and urine; however, its metabolites thymol sulphate and glucuronide were found and excreted in urine, and sulphate was also detected in plasma. Thalhamer et al. [62] detected metabolite p-cymene-2,5-diol and its oxidised form (p-cymene-2,5-dione) as the main products after a single oral administration of 50 mg of thymol to humans. The authors showed that human metabolism leads to the preferred hydroxylation of the aromatic system of thymol. In comparison with the results of Austgulen et al. [60], they found that some of the metabolites that were found in rat metabolism (p-cymene-3,9-diol and p-cymene-3,7-diol) could not be detected in human samples and vice versa (p-cymene-2,3-diol and p-cymene-3,8-diol detected in human samples). For this reason, future studies of thymol metabolism in different species of vertebrates are necessary [63]. Michiels et al. [64] demonstrated that the absorption of thymol in piglets was intensive in the stomach and the proximal segments of the small intestine, and they also found rapid renal excretion of free and conjugated thymol. With the detected percentage of intake recovered in bile determined to be 4.1%, they showed that enterohepatic recycling cannot be neglected. Thymol concentrations have also been detected in the plasma, milk, liver, kidney and fat of cattle after intramammary administration of a herbal product containing the essential oil of *Thymus vulgaris* [65,66]. According to the studies of Kohlert et al. [55], Rubió et al. [67] and Rubió et al. [68], the free form of thymol could not be detected in plasma, but thymol conjugates originating from biotransformation in humans and animals were detected. Thymol glucuronide was found for the first time in rat plasma after a single oral dose of 1.5 g of thyme extract to animals, containing 44.32 µM of thymol [68]. The presence of thymol in blood plasma after enzymatic cleavage of the conjugates was detected in the plasma of horses after the administration of Bronchipret® TP tablets with a thymol content of about 15 mg (the thymol concentration in plasma ranged from 62.4 to 315.9 ng/mL) by Van den Hoven et al. [69]. Haselmeyer et al. [70] detected thymol in broiler chickens fed with thyme herb (thymol concentrations in feed were 5–55 mg/kg). They found that thymol was quantified in the small intestine (115.5–1289.5 ng/g DM), the caecum (101.2–663.1 ng/g DM) and plasma (47.3–412.2 ng/mL), and it was only detected at the highest doses following enzymatic cleavage in the muscle and liver. However, the levels detected were relatively low. Haselmeyer [71] investigated the absorption of different thymol concentrations (2, 10 and 20 ug/mL) through the small intestine mucosa using the ex vivo method and Ussing chambers. He found that thymol concentrations in the mucosa/submucosa reached 7.5, 9.9 and 8.45% from the initial concentrations. Zitterl-Eglseer et al. [72] fed piglets with Biomin® P.E.P 1000 feed additive (essential oil blended from oregano, anise and citrus peels; the main compounds thymol and carvacrol) and detected thymol at a low concentration in plasma (15.4 ng/mL), kidney (23.4 ng/g) and faeces (24.4 ng/g). In the study conducted by Hagmuller et al. [73], *Thymi herba* was given as a feed additive to weanling piglets at different concentrations (0.1, 0.5 and 1%). Thymol was detectable in all plasma samples, and the thymol level increased with greater amounts of thyme herbs. Fernandez et al. [74] validated for the first time an analytical extraction procedure (a headspace solid-phase microextraction technique followed by gas chromatography/mass spectrometry) as a method to detect and quantify thymol in the faeces and egg yolk of Japanese quail.

The thymol concentrations in the plasma, duodenal wall, liver, kidney, breast muscle and content of all the intestinal segments of broiler chickens were analysed after 4 weeks of consumption of thyme essential oil by Oceľová [63] and Oceľová et al. [75]. Thymol was determined through the length of the intestinal tract for the first time in these studies, and the results obtained pointed to intensive thymol absorption in the proximal part of the small intestine. They detected 37% of the thymol duodenal content in the duodenal wall, which confirmed its efficient absorption from the intestinal tract. The authors pointed to intensive metabolism in the liver and the subsequent transport of thymol to the kidneys, as the thymol concentration detected in the liver was 11 times lower than in the kidney. The lowest concentration of thymol was detected in muscle tissue. Pisarčíková et al. [76] focused their attention on detecting the two main thymol metabolites of the second phase of biotransformation processes, thymol sulphate and glucuronide in plasma, in the duodenal wall and liver. Thymol sulphate was detected at all levels of thyme essential oil addition (0.01, 0.05 and 0.1%), and the highest concentration was found in the duodenal wall, with the lowest in the liver. Thymol glucuronide was only detected in all biological samples at the highest thyme essential oil concentration (0.1%).

The small number of these studies indicates that there is insufficient information about thymol distribution in animal and human tissues despite the fact that the beneficial effect of thymol depends on its absorption and accumulation in the organism. In this section, we summarised the current knowledge of thymol and its metabolite deposition in different tissues.

Table 1. Detection of thymol and its metabolites in the bodies of humans and animals.

| Animal Species | Applied Form | Detectable Compounds | Samples | References |
|---|---|---|---|---|
| human | thymol/orally | thymol glucuronide thymol sulphate thymohydroquinone sulphate thymol | urine | [59] |
| human | Bronchipret® TP/orally (equivalent to 1.08 mg thymol) | thymol sulphate | plasma, urine | [55] |
| | | thymol glucuronide | urine | |
| human | thymol/orally | p-cymene-2,5-diol p-cymene-2,3-diol p-cymene-3-ol-8-ene | urine | [62] |
| human | dried thyme/orally | thymol sulphate caffeic acid sulphate hydroxyphenylpropionic acid sulphate | plasma | [67] |

Table 1. Cont.

| Animal Species | Applied Form | Detectable Compounds | Samples | References |
|---|---|---|---|---|
| | | thymol sulphate caffeic acid sulphate hydroxyphenylpropionic acid sulphate thymol glucuronide | urine | |
| rabbit | thymol/orally | glucuronic acid ethereal sulphuric acid thymol | urine | [59] |
| rabbit | thymol/orally | thymol | plasma, small intestinal wall, liver, kidney, spleen, caecum, colon, muscle, faeces | [58] |
| rat | thymol/orally | p-cymene-2,5-diol p-cymene-3,9-diol p-cymene-3,7-diol thymol | urine | [60] |
| rat | thyme extract/orally | thymol sulphate | plasma | [68] |
| laying hen | thyme extract/orally | p-cymene-2,3-diol thymol | egg yolk | [61] |
| Japanese quail | thymol/orally | thymol | egg yolk, faeces | [74] |
| broiler chicken | dried *Thymi herba*/orally | thymol | plasma, small intestine, caecum, liver, muscle | [70] |
| broiler chicken | thyme essential oil/orally | thymol | plasma, liver, kidney, muscle, duodenal wall, gut content | [63] |
| broiler chicken | thyme essential oil/orally | thymol sulphate thymol glucuronide | plasma, duodenal wall, liver | [76] |
| piglet | essential oil/orally (carvacrol, thymol, eugenol and trans-cinnamaldehyde) | carvacrol thymol eugenol | plasma | [64] |
| | | carvacrol thymol eugenol trans-cinnamaldehyde | small intestine | |
| | | carvacrol thymol eugenol trans-cinnamaldehyde | bile | |
| | | carvacrol thymol eugenol | urine | |
| piglet | Biomin® P.E.P 1000 (main compounds thymol and carvacrol)/orally | thymol | plasma, kidney, faeces | [72] |

Table 1. *Cont.*

| Animal Species | Applied Form | Detectable Compounds | Samples | References |
|---|---|---|---|---|
| piglet | *Thymi herba*/orally | thymol | plasma | [73] |
| bovine | Phyto-Mast (essential oil of *Thymus vulgaris* and oregano)/intramammary | thymol | milk, plasma, liver, kidney, fat | [65] |
| dairy cattle | Phyto-Mast (essential oil of *Thymus vulgaris* and oregano)/intramammary | thymol | milk, plasma, liver, kidney, fat | [66] |
| horse | Bronchipret (equivalent to 2–4 g thyme extract)/orally | thymol | plasma | [69] |

## 3. Bioavailability of Thymol Generally and in Rabbits as Model Animal

To describe the metabolic processes of thymol in an organism, we chose the rabbit as a model animal because it represents an appropriate model for the evaluation of the bioavailability of nutrients. Phytogenic compounds and other foreign substances after oral administration are absorbed from the intestine, metabolised and eliminated from the organism. Once they reach the intestine or liver, they are converted during biotransformation processes (phase I and phase II) to more hydrophilic forms, and their pharmacological properties usually differ compared to the parental compound. It is also important to emphasise that metabolites can probably be deconjugated to the parental compound and express their pharmacological activity in this way. The major reactions occurring during phase I are oxidation, reduction and hydrolysis; phase II reactions are also called conjugation reactions and include glucuronidation, sulphation, acetylation, methylation, conjugation with glutathione and conjugation with amino acids [77–82].

The intestine plays an important role as a site for the absorption as well as biotransformation of thymol [63,76]. Thymol or its metabolites, after biotransformation processes in the intestinal wall, can be transported back into the intestinal lumen or are converted back to the parental compounds and redistributed within the organism through the systemic circulation [78]. Some part of the compounds are transported by the mesenteric vein into the liver, where they are metabolised, excreted into the duodenum in bile and again reabsorbed [57,78]. Bacova et al. [58] found 15% of thymol in the liver compared with the intestinal wall, which demonstrates the intensive absorption of thymol from the intestinal wall through the vena portae to the liver.

Oceľová [63] and Bacova et al. [58] detected significantly higher levels of thymol in the kidney in comparison with the liver and plasma, which shows that, although the liver is the most important organ where biotransformation processes occur, kidney microsomes are probably more effective. Kohlert et al. [55] showed that thymol metabolites are able to be reabsorbed in the proximal part of the kidney tubule, are cleaved by enzymes located in the brush border and are again reabsorbed.

There are some barriers that the compounds must pass through during their metabolic path in the organism, and they limit their absorption [63,79]. The first-pass metabolism in the intestine decreases the number of molecules reaching the blood circulation, and then the first-pass metabolism in the liver represents another barrier for the distribution of compounds in the organism. In addition to this, many efflux transporters are bound mainly with lipophilic molecules, which are rapidly excreted from the organism, greatly limiting their bioavailability [58,78,80–82]. These biotransformation processes are probably the reason why only a trace amount of thymol is found in the muscle and fat tissues of broilers [70,77] and rabbits [58].

The rabbit's digestive processes represent a complex system of the separation of digestible and indigestible parts of ingested food in the proximal colon [83]. The most important mechanism by which nutrients are released from ingested food is microbial fermentation in the caecum. The products of fermentation are either absorbed directly through the caecal wall or are re-ingested as caecotrophs [84]. The caecum and colon are the most important parts of a rabbit's digestive system in connection with the original feature of digestion, caecotrophy. Bacova et al. [57], Bacova et al. [58] and Placha et al. [85], after thymol addition to a rabbit's diet for 21 days and after its withdrawal from feed for the next 7 days, found a 6 times (7 times after withdrawal) higher concentration in plasma than in the intestinal wall. The authors attribute this finding to the metabolic processes that are present mainly in the caecum and that are responsible for the amount of thymol in caecotrophs. They stated that the mucus that covers the caecotrophs protects them, that the processes of fermentation continue until they reach the intestine and that thymol could be released and again reabsorbed into systemic circulation. The authors showed that, even though thymol was withdrawn, the metabolic processes of thymol were active, which was probably the consequence of caecotrophy.

Studying thymol bioavailability in different tissues is essential to understand its mechanism of action in target organs in which it can exert its biological role. Oral bioavailability represents the fraction of administered thymol reaching the systemic circulation and is a key parameter that affects its efficacy. Therefore, to propose an appropriate dose, the study of its oral bioavailability has received significant attention. However, only a few studies on thymol oral bioavailability have been carried out to date.

The organ bioavailability barriers to thymol are depicted in Figure 1.

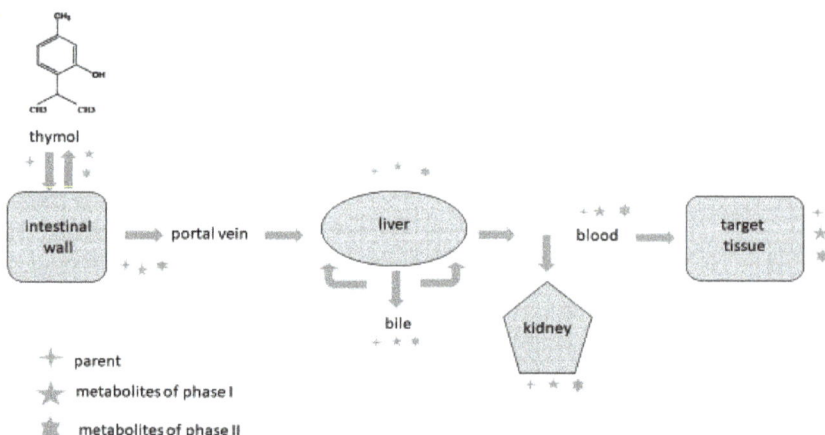

Figure 1. Organ bioavailability barriers to thymol (based on [79]).

## 4. Conclusions

In conclusion, this literature review reports the future perspectives of modern thymol application in humans and animals. This review summarises the available literature on thymol application as a feed additive in humans and animals, with emphasis on its metabolic route and oral bioavailability. The presented data represent the available scientific information regarding the urgent need for more studies to precisely understand the metabolic processes and biological activity of thymol and its metabolites within organisms. This information will be useful for researchers, drug and pharmaceutical industries and the medical and veterinary sectors.

**Author Contributions:** Writing—original draft preparation: I.P.; writing—review and editing: K.B. and L.P. All authors have read and agreed to the published version of the manuscript and agree to be accountable for its contents.

**Funding:** This research was funded by the Scientific Grant Agency of the Ministry for Education, Science, Research and Sport of the Slovak Republic and the Slovak Academy of Sciences (VEGA 2/0009/20).

**Informed Consent Statement:** Not applicable.

**Data Availability Statement:** The study did not report any data.

**Acknowledgments:** The authors thank to native English language editor, David McLean for improving the written English of the manuscript.

**Conflicts of Interest:** The authors declare no conflict of interest.

# References

1. Giacometti, J.; Kovacevic, D.B.; Putnik, P.; Gabric, D.; Bilusic, T.; Kresic, G.; Stulic, V.; Barba, F.J.; Chemat, F.; Barbosa-Canovas, G.; et al. Extraction of bioactive compounds and essential oils from Mediterranesn herbs by conventional and green innovative techniques: A review. *Food. Res. Int.* **2018**, *113*, 245–262. [CrossRef] [PubMed]
2. Oliveira, M.S.; Almeida, M.M.; Salazar, M.L.A.R.; Pires, F.C.S.; Bezzera, F.W.F.; Cunha, V.M.B.; Cordeiro, R.M.; Urbina, G.R.O.; Silva, A.P.S.; Pinto, R.H.H.; et al. Potential of medicinal use of essential oils from aromatic plants. In *Potential of Essential Oils*; El-Shemy, H., Ed.; IntechOpen: London, UK, 2018; pp. 1–19. [CrossRef]
3. Schmidt, B.; Ribnicky, D.M.; Poulev, A.; Logendra, S.; Cefalu, W.T.; Raskin, I. A natural history of botanical therapeutics. *Metab. Clin. Exp.* **2008**, *57* (Suppl. S1), S3–S9. [CrossRef] [PubMed]
4. Giannenas, I.; Sidiropoulou, E.; Bonos, E.; Christaki, E.; Florou-Paneri, P. The history of herbs, medicinal and aromatic plants, and their extracts: Past, current situation and future perspectives. In *Feed Additives, Aromatic Plants and Herbs in Animal Nutrition and Health*; Florou-Paneri, P., Christaki, E., Giannenas, I., Eds.; Elsevier Academic Press, Inc.: London, UK, 2020; pp. 1–15.
5. Genser, D. Food and drug Interaction: Consequences for the nutrition/health status. *Ann. Nutr. Metab.* **2008**, *52* (Suppl. S1), 29–32. [CrossRef] [PubMed]
6. Ribeiro dos Santos, R.; Andrade, M.; Sanches-Silva, A.; De Melo, N.R. Essential oils for food application: Natural substances with established biological activities. *Food Bioprocess. Technol.* **2017**, *11*, 43–71. [CrossRef]
7. Brown, E.D.; Wright, G.D. Antibacterial drugs discovery in the resistance era. *Nature* **2016**, *529*, 336–343. [CrossRef]
8. Atanasov, A.G.; Waltenberger, B.; Pferschy-Wenzig, E.M.; Linder, T.; Wawrosch, C.; Uhrin, P.; Temml, V.; Wang, L.; Schwaiger, S.; Heiss, E.H.; et al. Discovery and resupply of pharmacologically active plant-derived natural products: A review. *Biotechnol. Adv.* **2015**, *33*, 1582–1614. [CrossRef]
9. Tortorella, E.; Tedesco, P.; Esposito, P.F.; January, G.G.; Fani, R.; Jaspars, M.; de Pascale, D. Antibiotics from deep-sea microorganisms: Current discoveries and perspectives. *Mar. Drugs* **2018**, *16*, 355. [CrossRef]
10. Penesyan, A.; Khelleberg, S.; Egan, S. Development of novel drugs from marine surface associated microorganisms. *Mar. Drugs* **2010**, *8*, 438–459. [CrossRef]
11. Chavan, S.S.; Damale, M.G.; Devanand, B.S.; Sangshetti, J.N. Antibacterial and antifungal drugs from natural source: A review of clinical development. *Nat. Prod. Clin. Trials* **2018**, *1*, 114–164. [CrossRef]
12. Boucher, H.W.; Ambrose, P.G.; Chambers, H.F.; Ebright, R.H.; Jezek, A.; Murray, B.E.; Newland, J.G.; Ostrowsky, B.; Rex, J.H. White paper: Developing antimicrobial drugs for resistane pathogens, narrow-spectrum indivations, and unmet needs. *J. Infect. Dis.* **2017**, *216*, 228–236. [CrossRef]
13. Chen, S.; Song, J.; Sun, C.; Xu, J.; Zhu, Y.; Verpoorte, R.; Fan, T.P. Herbal genomics: Examining the biology of traditional medicines. *Science* **2015**, *347*, S27–S29. [CrossRef]
14. Newman, D.J.; Cragg, G.M. Natural products as sources of new drugs from 1981 to 2014. *J. Nat. Prod.* **2016**, *79*, 629–661. [CrossRef] [PubMed]
15. Anand, U.; Jacobo-Herrera, N.; Altemimi, A.; Lakhssassi, N. A comprehensive review on medicicnal plants as antimicrobial therapeutics: Potential avenues of biocompatible grug discovery. *Metabolites* **2019**, *9*, 258. [CrossRef] [PubMed]
16. Raskin, I.; Ribnicky, D.M.; Komarnytsky, S.; Ilic, N.; Poulev, A.; Borisjuk, N.; Brinker, A.; Moreno, D.A.; Ripoll, C.; Yakoby, N.; et al. Plants and human health in the twenty-first century. *Trends Biotechnol.* **2002**, *20*, 522–531. [CrossRef]
17. European Medicines Agency (EMA) 2014. Sales of Veterinary Antimicrobial Agents in 26 EU/EEA Countries in 2012. Available online: http://www.ema.europa.eu/docs/enGB/document_libraryReport/2014/10/WC500175671.pdf (accessed on 1 March 2022).
18. Federal Food Safety and Veterinary Office 2019. Statistics and Reports. Swiss Antibiotic Resistance Report 2018. Available online: www.blv.admin.ch/blv/en/home/tiere/publikationen-und-forschung/statistiken-berichte-tiere (accessed on 1 March 2022).
19. Bennett, R.M.; Christiansen, K.; Clifton-Hadley, R.S. Direct costs of endemic diseases of farm animals in Great Britain. *Vet. Rec.* **1999**, *145*, 376–377. [CrossRef]

20. Bradley, A. Bovine mastitis: An evolving disease. *Vet. J.* **2002**, *164*, 116–128. [CrossRef]
21. Mertenat, D.; Dal Cero, M.; Vogl, C.R.; Ivemeyer, S.; Meier, B.; Maeschli, A.; Hamburger, M.; Walkenhorst, M. Ethnoveterinary knowledge of farmers in bilingual regions of Switzerland – is there potential to extend veterinary options to reduce antimicrobial use? *J. Ethnopharmacol.* **2020**, *246*, 112184. [CrossRef]
22. Woolhouse, M.; Ward, M.; van Bunnik, B.; Farrar, J. Antimicrobial resistance in humans, livestock and the wider environment. *Philos. Trans. R. Soc. Lond. B Biol. Sci.* **2015**, *370*, 1670. [CrossRef]
23. Second Joint FAO/OIE/WHO Expert Workshop on Non-human Antimicrobial Usage and Antimicrobial Resistance: Management Options, Oslo, Norway, 15–18 March 2004. Available online: www.oie.int/doc/ged/D895.PDF (accessed on 1 March 2022).
24. Marshall, B.M.; Levy, S.B. Food animals and antimicrobials: Impacts on human health. *Clin. Microbiol. Rev.* **2011**, *24*, 718–733. [CrossRef]
25. Maeschli, A.; Schmidt, A.; Ammann, W.; Schurtenberger, P.; Maurer, E.; Walkenhorst, M. Einfluss eines komplementarmedizinischen telefonischen Beratungssystems auf den Antibiotikaeinsatz bei Nutztieren in der Schweiz. *Complement. Med. Res.* **2019**, *26*, 174–181. [CrossRef]
26. Ayrle, H.; Mevissen, M.; Kaske, M.; Nathues, H.; Grutzner, N.; Melzig, M.; Walkenhorst, M. Medicinal plants – prophylactic and therapeutic options for gastrointestinal and respiratory diseases in calves and piglets? A systematic review. *BMC Vet. Res.* **2016**, *12*, 89. [CrossRef] [PubMed]
27. Kupper, J.; Walkenhorst, M.; Ayrle, H.; Mevissen, M.; Demuth, D.; Naegeli, H. Online-Informationssystem für die Phytotherapie bei Tieren. *Schweiz. Arch. Tierheilkd.* **2018**, *10*, 589–595. [CrossRef] [PubMed]
28. Lou, S.N.; Hsu, Y.S.; Ho, C.T. Flavonoid compositions and antioxidant activity of calamondin extracts prepared using different solvents. *J. Food Drug Anal.* **2014**, *22*, 290–295. [CrossRef]
29. Do, Q.D.; Angkawijaya, A.E.; Tran-Nguyen, P.L.; Huynh, L.H.; Soetaredjo, F.E.; Ismadji, S.; Ju, Y.H. Effect of extraction solvent on total phenol content, total flavonoid content, and antioxidant activity of *Limnophila aromatica*. *J. Food Drug Anal.* **2014**, *22*, 296–302. [CrossRef]
30. Yu, Y.M.; Chao, T.Y.; Chang, W.C.; Chang, M.J.; Lee, M.F. Thymol reduces oxidative stress, aortic intimal thickening, and inflammation-related gene expression in hyperlipidemic rabbits. *J. Food Drug Anal.* **2016**, *24*, 556–563. [CrossRef]
31. Meeran, M.F.N.; Javed, H.; Taee, H.A.; Azimullah, S.; Ojha, S.K. Pharmacological properties and molecular mechanisms of thymol: Prospects for its therapeutic potential and pharmaceutical development. *Front. Pharmacol.* **2017**, *8*, 380. [CrossRef] [PubMed]
32. Castillo-España, P.; Cisneros-Estrada, A.; Garduno-Ramirez, M.L.; Hernandez-Abreu, O.; Ramirez, R.; Estrada-Soto, S. Preliminary ethnopharmacological survey of plants used in Mexico for the treatment of hypertension. *Phcog. Rev.* **2009**, *3*, 41–65. [CrossRef]
33. Giordani, R.; Hadef, Y.; Kaloustian, J. Compositions and antifungal activities of essential oils of some Algerian aromatic plants. *Fitoterapia* **2008**, *79*, 199–203. [CrossRef] [PubMed]
34. Al-Bayati, F.A. Synergistic antibacterial activity between *Thymus vulgaris* and *Pimpinella anisum* essential oils and methanol extracts. *J. Ethnophamacol.* **2008**, *116*, 403–406. [CrossRef]
35. Nikolić, M.; Glamočlija, J.; Ferreira, I.C.F.R.; Calheha, R.; Fernandes, A.; Markovič, T.; Markovič, D.; Giweli, A.; Sokovič, M. Chemical composition, antimicrobial, antioxidant and antitumor activity of *Thymus serpyllum* L., *Thymus algeriensis* Boiss. and Reut and *Thymus vulgaris* L. essential oils. *Ind. Cros. Prod.* **2014**, *52*, 183–190. [CrossRef]
36. Roth, G.A.; Forouzanfar, M.H.; Moran, A.E.; Barber, R.; Nguyen, G.; Feigin, V.L.; Naghavi, M.; Mensah, G.A.; Murray, C.J.L.; Phil, D. Demographic and epidemiologic drivers of global cardiovascular mortality. *N. Engl. J. Med.* **2015**, *372*, 1333–1341. [CrossRef]
37. Chang, X.; Zhang, T.; Zhang, W.; Zhao, Z.; Sun, J. Natural drugs a treatment strategy for cardiovascular disease through the regulation of oxidative stress. *Oxid. Med. Cell. Longev.* **2020**, *2020*, 5430407. [CrossRef]
38. Senoner, T.; Dichtl, W. Oxidative stress in cardiovascular diseases: Still a therapeutic target? *Nutrient* **2019**, *11*, 2090. [CrossRef]
39. Costa, G.; Fortuna, A.; Gonçalves, D.; Figueiredo, I.V.; Falcão, A.; Batista, M.T. Pharmacokinetics of *Cymbopogon citratus* infusion in rats after single oral dose administration. *SOJ Pharm. Pharm. Sci.* **2017**, *4*, 1–9. [CrossRef]
40. Suen, J.; Thomas, J.; Kranz, A.; Vun, S.; Miller, M. Effect of flavonoids on oxidative stress and inflammation in adults at risk of cardiovascular disease: A systematic review. *Healthcare* **2016**, *4*, 69. [CrossRef] [PubMed]
41. Al-Rawi, N.H.; Shahid, A.M. Oxidative stress, antioxidants, and lipid profile in the serum and saliva of individuals with coronary heart disease: Is there a link with periodontal health? *Minerva Stomatol.* **2017**, *66*, 212–225. [CrossRef]
42. Pignatelli, P.; Menichelli, D.; Pastori, D.; Violi, F. Oxidative stress and cardiovascular disease: New insights. *Kardiol. Pol.* **2018**, *76*, 713–722. [CrossRef] [PubMed]
43. Harrison, D.; Griendling, K.K.; Landmesser, U.; Hornig, B.; Drexler, H. Role of oxidative stress in atherosclerosis. *Am. J. Cardiol.* **2003**, *91*, 7A–11A. [CrossRef]
44. de Brito Alves, J.L.; de Sousa, V.P.; Cavalcanti Neto, M.P.; Magnani, M.; de Andrade Braga, V.; da Costa-Silva, J.H.; Leandro, C.G.; Vidal, H.; Pirola, L. New insights on the use of dietary polyphenols or probiotics for the management of arterial hypertension. *Front. Physiol.* **2016**, *7*, 448. [CrossRef]
45. Selma, M.V.; Espín, J.C.; Tomás-Barberán, F.A. Interaction between phenolics and gut microbiota: Role in human health. *J. Agric. Food Chem.* **2009**, *57*, 6485–6501. [CrossRef]
46. Tomas-Barberan, F.A.; Selma, M.V.; Espin, J.C. Interactions of gut microbiota with dietary polyphenols and consequences to human health. *Curr. Opin. Clin. Nutr. Metab. Care* **2016**, *19*, 471–476. [CrossRef] [PubMed]

47. Natarajan, N.; Hori, D.; Flavahan, S.; Steppan, J.; Flavahan, N.A.; Berkowitz, D.E.; Pluznick, J.L. Microbial short chain fatty acid metabolites lower blood pressure via endothelial G protein-coupled receptor 41. *Physiol. Genom.* **2016**, *48*, 826–834. [CrossRef] [PubMed]
48. Calderón-Pérez, L.; Gosalbes, M.J.; Yuste, S.; Valls, R.M.; Pedret, A.; Llauradó, E.; Jimenez-Hernandez, N.; Artacho, A.; Pla-Paga, L.; Companys, J.; et al. Gut metagenomic and short chain fatty acids signature in hypertension: A cross-sectional study. *Sci. Rep.* **2020**, *10*, 6436. [CrossRef] [PubMed]
49. Calderon-Pérez, L.; Llauradó, E.; Companys, J.; Pla-Paga, L.; Pedret, A.; Rubió, L.; Gosalbes, M.J.; Yuste, S.; Sola, R.; Valls, R.M. Interplay between dietary phenolic compound intake and the human gut microbiome in hypertension: A cross-sectional study. *Food Chem.* **2021**, *344*, 128567. [CrossRef]
50. Salehi, B.; Mishra, A.P.; Shukla, I.; Sharifi-Rad, M.; Contreras, M.D.M.; Segura-Carretero, A.; Fathi, H.; Nasrabadi, N.N.; Kobarfard, F.; Sharifi-Rad, J. Thymol, thyme, and other plant sources: Health and potential uses. *Phytother. Res.* **2018**, *32*, 1688–1706. [CrossRef]
51. Komaki, A.; Hoseini, F.; Shahidi, S.; Baharlouei, H. Study of the effect of extract of *Thymus vulgaris* on anxiety in male rats. *J. Tradit. Complem. Med.* **2016**, *6*, 257–261. [CrossRef]
52. Asadbegi, M.; Yaghmaei, P.; Salehi, I.; Komaki, A.; Ebrahim-Habibi, A. Investigation of thymol effect on learning and memory impairment induced by intrahippocampal injection of amyloid beta peptide in high fat diet-fed rats. *Metab. Brain Dis.* **2017**, *32*, 827–839. [CrossRef]
53. Kohlert, C.; van Rensen, I.; März, R.; Schindler, G.; Graefe, E.U.; Veit, M. Bioavailability and pharmacokinetics of natural volatile terpenes in animals and humans. *Planta Med.* **2000**, *66*, 495–505. [CrossRef]
54. Rubió, L.; Macià, A.; Castell-Auví, A.; Pinent, M.; Blay, M.T.; Ardévol, A.; Romero, M.P.; Motilva, M.J. Effect of the co-occurring olive oil and thyme extracts on the phenolic bioaccessibility and bioavailability assessed by in vitro digestion and cell models. *Food Chem.* **2014**, *149*, 277–284. [CrossRef]
55. Kohlert, C.; Schindler, G.; März, R.W.; Abel, G.; Brinkhaus, B.; Derendorf, H.; Gräfe, E.U.; Veit, M. Systemic availability and pharmacokinetics of thymol in humans. *J. Clin. Pharmacol.* **2002**, *42*, 731–737. [CrossRef]
56. Thomford, N.E.; Senthebane, D.A.; Rowe, A.; Munro, D.; Seele, P.; Maroyi, A.; Dzobo, K. Natural products for drug discovery in the 21st century: Innovations for novel drug discovery. *Int. J. Mol. Sci.* **2018**, *19*, 1578. [CrossRef] [PubMed]
57. Bacova, K.; Zitterl-Eglseer, K.; Chrastinova, L.; Laukova, A.; Madarova, M.; Gancarcikova, S.; Sopkova, D.; Andrejcakova, Z.; Placha, I. Effect of thymol addition and withdrawal on some blood parameters, antioxidative defence system and fatty acid profile in rabbit muscle. *Animals* **2020**, *10*, 1248. [CrossRef] [PubMed]
58. Bacova, K.; Zitterl Eglseer, K.; Karas Räuber, G.; Chrastinova, L.; Laukova, A.; Takacsova, M.; Pogany Simonova, M.; Placha, I. Effect of sustained administration of thymol on its bioaccessibility and bioavailability in rabbits. *Animals* **2021**, *11*, 2595. [CrossRef] [PubMed]
59. Takada, M.; Agata, I.; Sakamoto, M.; Yagi, N.; Hayashi, N. On the metabolic detoxication of thymol in rabbit and man. *J. Toxicol. Sci.* **1979**, *4*, 341–350. [CrossRef] [PubMed]
60. Austgulen, L.; Solheim, E.; Scheline, R. Metabolism in rats of p-cymene derivatives: Carvacrol and thymol. *Pharmacol. Toxicol.* **1987**, *61*, 98–102. [CrossRef]
61. Krause, E.L.; Ternes, W. Bioavailability of the antioxidative thyme compounds thymol and p-cymene-2,3-diol in egg. *Eur. Food Res. Technol.* **1999**, *209*, 140–144. [CrossRef]
62. Thalhamer, B.; Buchberger, W.; Waser, M. Identification of thymol phase I metabolites in human urine by headspace sorptive extraction combined with thermal desorption and gas chromatography mass spectrometry. *J. Pharm. Biomed. Anal.* **2011**, *56*, 64–69. [CrossRef]
63. Oceľová, V. Plant additives in relation to the animal gastrointestinal tract and metabolism of their main compounds. Master's Thesis, Institute of Animal Physiology, Slovak Academy of Sciences, Košice, Slovakia, 2017.
64. Michiels, J.; Missotten, J.; Dierick, N.; Fremaut, D.; Maene, P.; De Smet, S. In vitro degradation and in vivo passage kinetics of carvacrol, thymol, eugenol and trans-cinnamaldehyde along the gastrointestinal tract of piglets. *J. Sci. Food Agric.* **2008**, *88*, 2371–2381. [CrossRef]
65. Armorini, S.; Yeatts, J.E.; Mullen, K.A.E.; Mason, S.E.; Mehmeti, E.; Anderson, K.L.; Washburn, S.P.; Baynes, R.E. Development of a HS-SPME-GC-MS/MS method for the quantitation of thymol and carvacrol in bovine matrices and to determine residue depletion in milk and tissues. *J. Agric. Food Chem.* **2016**, *64*, 7856–7865. [CrossRef]
66. Mason, S.E.; Mullen, K.A.E.; Anderson, K.L.; Washburn, S.P.; Yeatts, J.L.; Baynes, R.E. Pharmacokinetic analysis of thymol, carvacrol and diallyl disulfide after intramammary and topical applications in healthy organic dairy cattle. *Food Addit. Contam. Part A* **2017**, *34*, 740–749. [CrossRef]
67. Rubió, L.; Farràs, M.; de la Torre, R.; Macià, A.; Romero, M.P.; Valls, R.M.; Solà, R.; Farré, M.; Fitó, M.; Motilva, M.J. Metabolite profiling of olive oil and thyme phenols after a sustained intake of two phenol-enriched olive oils by humans: Identification of compliance markers. *Food Res. Int.* **2014**, *65*, 59–68. [CrossRef]
68. Rubió, L.; Serra, A.; Chen, C.Y.O.; Macià, A.; Romero, M.P.; Covas, M.I.; Solà, R.; Motilva, M.J. Effects of co-occurring components from olive oil and thyme extracts on antioxidant status and their bioavailability in acute ingestion in rats. *Food Funct.* **2014**, *5*, 740–747. [CrossRef] [PubMed]

69. Van den Hoven, R.; Zappe, H.; Zitterl-Eglseer, K.; Jugl, M.; Franz, C. Study of the effect of Bronchipret on the lung function of five Austrian saddle horses suffering recurrent airway obstruction (heaves). *Vet. Rec.* **2003**, *152*, 555–557. [CrossRef] [PubMed]
70. Haselmeyer, A.; Zentek, J.; Chizzola, R. Effects of thyme as a feed additive in broiler chickens on thymol in gut contents, blood plasma, liver and muscle. *J. Sci. Food Agric.* **2015**, *95*, 504–508. [CrossRef] [PubMed]
71. Haselmeyer, A. Wirkung von Thymian als Futterzusatz beim Broiler. Ph.D. Thesis, Veterinärmedizinischen Universität, Wien, Austria, 2007.
72. Zitterl-Eglseer, K.; Wetscherek, W.; Stoni, A.; Kroismayr, A.; Windisch, W. Bioavailability of essential oils of a phytobiotic feed additive and impact of performance and nutrient digestibility in weaned piglets. *Bodenkult. J. Land Manag. Food Environ.* **2008**, *59*, 121–129.
73. Hagmüller, W.; Jugl-Chizzola, M.; Zitterl-Eglseer, K.; Gabler, C.; Spergser, J.; Chizzola, R.; Franz, C. The use of Thymi Herba as feed additive (0.1%, 0.5%, 1.0%) in weanling piglets with assessment of the shedding of haemolysing E. coli and the detection of thymol in the blood plasma. *Berl. Münch. Tierärztl. Wochenschr.* **2005**, *119*, 50–54.
74. Fernandez, M.E.; Palacio, M.A.; Labaque, M.C. Thymol detection by solid-phase microextraction in faeces and egg yolk of Japanese quail. *J. Chromatogr. B* **2017**, *1044*, 39–46. [CrossRef]
75. Oceľová, V.; Chizzola, R.; Battelli, G.; Pisarcikova, J.; Faix, S.; Gai, F.; Placha, I. Thymol in the intestinal tract of broiler chickens after sustained administration of thyme essential oil in feed. *J. Anim. Physiol. Anim. Nutr.* **2019**, *103*, 204–209. [CrossRef]
76. Pisarčíková, J.; Oceľová, V.; Faix, Š.; Plachá, I.; Calderón, A.I. Identification and quantification of thymol metabolites in plasma, liver and duodenal wall of broiler chickens using UHPLC-ESI-QTOF-MS. *Biomed. Chromatogr.* **2017**, *31*, e3881. [CrossRef]
77. Oceľová, V.; Chizzola, R.; Pisarčíková, J.; Novak, J.; Ivanišinová, O.; Faix, Š. Effect of thyme essential oil supplementation on thymol content in blood plasma, liver, kidney and muscle in broiler chickens. *Nat. Prod. Commun.* **2016**, *11*, 1545–1550. [CrossRef]
78. Singh, R.; Hu, M. Drug metabolism in gastrointestinal tract. In *Oral Bioavailability: Basic Principles, Advanced Concepts, and Applications*; Hu, M., Li, X., Eds.; John Wiley & Sons, Inc.: Hoboken, NJ, USA, 2011; pp. 91–109.
79. Hu, M.; Li, X. Barriers to oral bioavailability-an overview. In *Oral Bioavailability: Basic Principles, Advanced Concepts, and Applications*; Hu, M., Li, X., Eds.; John Wiley & Sons, Inc.: Hoboken, NJ, USA, 2011; pp. 1–5.
80. Parkinson, A. Biotransformation of Xenobiotics. In *Cassaret & Doull's Toxicology: The Basic Science of Poisons*, 6th ed.; Klaassen, C.D., Ed.; The McGraw-Hill Companies: New York, NY, USA, 2001; pp. 133–224.
81. Rozman, K.K.; Klaassen, C.D. Absorption, distribution, and excretion of toxicants. In *Cassaret & Doull's Toxicology: The Basic Science of Poisons*, 6th ed.; Klaassen, C.D., Ed.; The McGraw-Hill Companies: New York, NY, USA, 2001; pp. 107–132.
82. Timbrell, J.A. *Factors Affecting Toxic Responses: Disposition. Principles of Biochemical Toxicology*, 4th ed.; Informa Healthcare USA, Inc.: New York, NY, USA, 2009; pp. 35–74.
83. Davies, R.R.; Davies, J.A.E.R. Rabbit gastrointestinal physiology. *Vet. Clin. North Am. Exot. Anim. Pract.* **2003**, *6*, 139–153. [CrossRef]
84. Campbell-Ward, M.L. Gastrointestinal physiology and nutrition. In *Ferrets, Rabbits, and Rodents: Clinical Medicine and Surgery*, 3rd ed.; Quesenberry, K.E., Carpenter, J.W., Eds.; Elsevier: Saint-Louis, MI, USA, 2012; pp. 183–192.
85. Placha, I.; Bacova, K.; Zitterl-Eglseer, K.; Laukova, A.; Chrastinova, L.; Madarova, M.; Zitnan, R.; Strkolcova, G. Thymol in fattening rabbit diet, its bioavailability and effects on intestinal morphology, microbiota from caecal content and immunity. *J. Anim. Physiol. Anim. Nutr.* **2021**, *106*, 368–377. [CrossRef] [PubMed]

MDPI
St. Alban-Anlage 66
4052 Basel
Switzerland
Tel. +41 61 683 77 34
Fax +41 61 302 89 18
www.mdpi.com

*Animals* Editorial Office
E-mail: animals@mdpi.com
www.mdpi.com/journal/animals

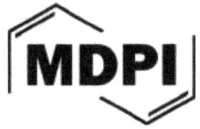

www.ingramcontent.com/pod-product-compliance
Lightning Source LLC
LaVergne TN
LVHW070552100526
838202LV00012B/448